ScrubTales™ Physical Therapist

A Real-World Career Guide That Tells the Truth About Rehabilitation, Productivity, and Outcomes

Mason Preddy

MMP
MASON MAISON
PUBLISHING™
REWRITING THE NARRATIVE
MASONMAISON.PUB

MASON MAISON
PUBLISHING™
REWRITING THE NARRATIVE
MASONMAISON.PUB

Published by Mason Maison™ Publishing (MMP)

healthcare career should carefully evaluate their personal circumstances, financial obligations, health considerations, and long-term professional goals before pursuing training or employment in the field.

The publisher and author disclaim any liability for loss, risk, or damages—whether direct, indirect, incidental, or consequential—arising from the use or application of the information presented in this publication.

Mason Maison™ Publishing (MMP) logo to appear on this page in final layout.

Chapter 1

A Note to the Reader: Understanding (gl) Terms

Throughout this book, you will occasionally see certain words followed by the notation **(gl)**. These markings indicate that the term appears in the Glossary at the back of the book, where you can find a clear, reader-friendly definition designed to help you quickly understand language that is commonly used in rehabilitation practice, healthcare systems, and professional training environments.

Healthcare has its own working vocabulary. Clinicians communicate using specialized terminology because precision improves safety, efficiency, and team coordination. For readers who are new to the profession—or who are exploring physical therapy as a future career—this language can initially feel unfamiliar. The **(gl)** markers are included to remove that barrier. Instead of interrupting the reading experience with long in-text explanations, key terms are tagged once at their first meaningful appearance so that you can reference them easily whenever needed.

You are not expected to memorize every glossary term immediately. Over time, repeated exposure to these concepts will make them feel natural, just as they do for practicing clinicians. The goal is not technical perfection; the goal is familiarity, confidence, and gradual fluency in the professional language you will encounter in classrooms, clinical training, and real-world rehabilitation settings.

If you ever come across a marked term and are unsure of its meaning, simply turn to the Glossary, review the definition, and return to the text. Each entry is written to be practical, concise, and directly relevant to the realities of physical therapy practice so that the learning process remains smooth, efficient, and grounded in everyday clinical use.

Chapter 2

Welcome & Introduction

Welcome to *ScrubTales™ Physical Therapist: A Real-World Career Guide That Tells the Truth About Rehabilitation, Productivity, and Outcomes.*

If you are holding this book, there is a strong possibility that you are considering a future in physical therapy, exploring a career transition, or trying to better understand what the profession truly looks like beyond admissions websites and promotional materials. Physical therapy is widely respected, deeply meaningful, and intellectually engaging work. It is also physically demanding, productivity-driven in many settings, and shaped heavily by reimbursement models, documentation requirements, and workplace structures that can significantly influence daily experience. Understanding both sides of that reality is essential before committing to the path.

The *ScrubTales™* series was created to present healthcare careers as they are actually lived rather than how they are often advertised. Instead of focusing only on education requirements, job descriptions, and salary averages, these guides explore workflow realities, emotional demands, team dynamics, compensation structures, long-term sustainability, and the alignment factors that determine whether a career energizes someone or slowly drains them. The goal is clarity. When readers clearly understand what a role asks of them — mentally, physically, emotionally, and operationally — they are able to make decisions that are intentional rather than reactive.

Throughout this book, you will meet members of the *SCRUBfits™**, a group of representative healthcare professionals who help interpret different aspects of the profession through multiple perspectives. Some will highlight the opportunities that make physical therapy deeply rewarding, while others will draw attention to the structural pressures that influence workload, productivity, and long-term career satisfaction. Their role is not to convince you to enter the profession; it is to help you see it more clearly so you can determine whether the path fits your goals, strengths, and long-range lifestyle priorities.

Healthcare careers shape more than work schedules. They influence financial trajectory, physical well-being, family routines, geographic mobility, emotional load, and long-term professional identity. Decisions of this scale deserve information that is honest, practical, and grounded in real-world experience. This guide is designed to provide that perspective — not to make the decision for you, but to ensure that whatever decision you make is informed, deliberate, and aligned.

In the pages ahead, you will encounter real-world career pathways, day-to-day clinical experiences, hiring intelligence, compensation realities, long-term career planning frameworks, and structured reflection tools designed to help you evaluate whether the profession of physical therapy truly fits you — before you commit.

Chapter 3

Why This Book Exists (and Why It Exists)

Most healthcare career guides are written to describe professions. This book was written to help you make a decision. There is an important difference between the two. Descriptions tell you what a profession is supposed to look like. Decision-support guidance helps you understand how a profession is actually experienced — day after day, year after year — so you can determine whether it aligns with how you naturally think, work, and live.

Many individuals choose healthcare careers based primarily on capability rather than alignment. Being capable of performing the work is not the same as being energized by the environment in which the work takes place. Physical therapy is widely respected, intellectually engaging, and deeply meaningful work that restores movement, independence, and quality of life for patients across a wide range of conditions. At the same time, the profession operates within real-world systems shaped by reimbursement structures, documentation requirements, scheduling intensity, productivity expectations, and workplace cultures that vary significantly across settings. These operational factors influence daily professional experience far more than most early career explorers are told. This book exists to make those realities visible before major educational, financial, and professional commitments are made.

Because the purpose of this guide is to support decision-making, it is designed to be flexible rather than strictly linear. Some readers begin with the Day-in-the-Life chapters to experience the rhythm of clinical work across different settings. Others start with the Fit Analyzer and reflection sections to evaluate whether the profession matches their personality, priorities, and long-term lifestyle preferences. Still others move directly to the hiring, compensation, and career navigation chapters to understand how early employment decisions shape long-term trajectory, workload sustainability, and financial outcomes. You may read the book in any order that best supports your exploration.

Throughout the manuscript, certain words include a (gl) marker, indicating that the term appears in the glossary for quick reference. Healthcare professions operate within specialized terminology that can initially feel unfamiliar, and early familiarity with these concepts helps reduce the cognitive load that many new clinicians experience when learning both professional language and clinical skills at the same time. The glossary is designed as a practical working reference rather than an academic vocabulary list, focusing on terms that appear frequently in real-world workflow, documentation, and interdisciplinary communication.

Approach this book as a mirror rather than a sales pitch. If the profession of physical therapy resonates with your strengths, interests, and preferred work style, the chapters ahead will help you prepare strategically and enter the field with clearer expectations. If certain aspects of the role feel misaligned, that information is equally valuable. Discovering alignment — or misalignment — early can save years of frustration, unnecessary debt, and difficult mid-career redirection. The goal of this guide is not to persuade you to become a physical therapist; it is to help you decide, with clarity and confidence, whether the path truly fits you.

Chapter 4

Who This Book Is For (and Who It Isn't)

This book is designed for individuals who are seriously exploring the profession of physical therapy and want an honest, real-world understanding of what the role demands before committing to the education, time, and financial investment required to enter the field. It is written for high school students beginning to explore healthcare careers, college students considering pre-physical therapy pathways, career changers evaluating a transition into rehabilitation professions, healthcare professionals considering a pivot into physical therapy, and practicing clinicians who want a clearer long-term roadmap for navigating the profession's evolving landscape.

It is also for readers who prefer decision clarity over career marketing. If you want to understand how productivity expectations influence daily schedules, how reimbursement systems shape treatment models, how workplace settings change workload intensity, and how career trajectory unfolds over five, ten, and twenty years, this guide is structured to help you evaluate those realities with transparency. Individuals who value alignment — matching their working style, energy patterns, physical capacity, and long-term lifestyle priorities to the demands of a profession — will find the reflection tools and decision frameworks especially useful.

At the same time, this book may not be the best fit for readers who are looking only for a brief overview of degree requirements, salary averages, or application checklists without deeper discussion of workplace realities and long-term career implications. While those topics are included, the focus of this guide is broader: helping you understand how the profession is actually experienced so you can make an informed, intentional decision rather than a rushed one.

You do not need to be certain that physical therapy is your final destination to benefit from this book. In fact, some readers discover through the reflection exercises and real-world insights that another healthcare path aligns more closely with their goals, interests, or lifestyle priorities. That outcome is not a failure of exploration; it is a success of informed decision-making. The purpose of this guide is not to convince you to choose physical therapy. Its purpose is to ensure that whichever path you ultimately choose is one that fits you.

Chapter 5

The Toll Booth™ — The Emotional, Cognitive, and Lifestyle Cost of Becoming a Physical Therapist

Every healthcare profession comes with rewards that are visible from the outside and costs that are often invisible until someone is living the work day after day. The *Toll Booth™* represents the cumulative emotional, cognitive, physical, and lifestyle demands that professionals pay over time in exchange for the opportunity to practice in their chosen field. Understanding these costs early does not discourage entry into a profession; it allows individuals to prepare realistically and determine whether the long-term tradeoffs align with how they want to live and work.

Physical therapy is deeply meaningful work centered on restoring movement, function, and independence. Clinicians often build strong patient relationships over weeks or months of treatment, witnessing measurable improvement that directly results from consistent therapeutic effort. These visible outcomes are one of the most energizing aspects of the profession. However, the daily experience of practice also includes operational pressures that shape workload and pace in ways that are not always discussed during early career exploration.

One of the primary cognitive demands of physical therapy practice involves maintaining continuous clinical decision-making across a high volume of patient encounters. Therapists must rapidly assess patient presentation, adapt treatment plans in real time, document progress accurately, and manage multiple active cases simultaneously while maintaining patient engagement and safety. Over time, the mental load of continuous clinical judgment combined with documentation requirements can become a significant contributor to professional fatigue if workflow systems or workplace structures do not adequately support clinicians.

Physical demands represent another component of the toll. Depending on the setting, therapists may spend long periods standing, transferring patients, demonstrating exercises, supporting mobility training, and performing repetitive movements throughout the day. While ergonomics awareness and physical conditioning can mitigate some of this strain, the profession still requires sustained physical engagement that accumulates across years of practice. Long-term musculoskeletal stress is an important factor to consider when evaluating career sustainability.

Productivity expectations also influence the lived experience of the profession. In many outpatient and rehabilitation environments, therapists operate within scheduling models designed to maintain high patient throughput. This can create tension between the desire to provide individualized care and the operational pressure to manage tightly scheduled treatment sessions while completing required documentation within limited administrative time. Learning to navigate productivity systems effectively is an essential professional skill that often determines whether clinicians feel in control of their workload or consistently behind it.

Lifestyle considerations extend beyond the clinic walls. Work schedules vary by setting, with some environments offering predictable daytime hours while others require evening appointments, rotating schedules, or weekend coverage depending on patient demand. Additionally, emotional investment in patient recovery — particularly when progress is slow or outcomes are uncertain — can contribute to emotional fatigue if clinicians do not develop effective boundary-setting and recovery strategies outside of work.

None of these factors diminish the value or impact of the profession. Instead, they represent the realistic operating conditions under which physical therapists practice. Many clinicians thrive in this environment, finding deep satisfaction in functional patient outcomes and long-term rehabilitation relationships. Others discover that certain practice settings align better with their preferred pace, workload structure, or lifestyle priorities. Understanding the *Toll Booth™* early allows individuals to make intentional choices about where and how they practice, transforming potential strain into manageable, planned tradeoffs rather than unexpected sources of burnout later in their careers.

Chapter 6

Meet the SCRUBfits™

Meet the SCRUB*fits*™ — Physical Therapy

Every healthcare profession carries more than a job description; it carries a rhythm. Some roles demand rapid decision-making and constant urgency, while others reward patience, persistence, and the ability to guide progress that unfolds over weeks or months rather than minutes. Physical therapy belongs to that second rhythm — a profession built on consistency, trust, and the ability to motivate people through recovery that is often slower than they wish and more difficult than they expected.

The **SCRUB*fits*™** exist to make these deeper professional rhythms visible. They are not mascots or personality labels. They are alignment archetypes — narrative guides representing the real ways clinicians think, communicate, pace their work, and sustain themselves across long healthcare careers. Each **SCRUB*fits*™** voice helps translate what the profession *feels like* from the inside, allowing you to evaluate not only whether you can perform the role, but whether the daily experience of the work aligns with how you naturally operate.

In the physical therapy journey, your primary guide is **Lilac Lift, DPT**. Lilac represents clinicians who thrive in environments where progress is built session by session, where encouragement is as important as technique, and where patient relationships often extend across weeks or months of care. Her reflections throughout this book are designed to help you interpret what the physical therapy profession truly asks of its practitioners — the physical stamina required, the emotional patience involved in long recoveries, the productivity expectations that shape daily schedules, and the habits that allow therapists to remain energized over time. Her goal is not to persuade you toward the profession, but to help you recognize whether the rhythm of physical therapy feels sustainable and meaningful for you.

Chapter 7

Day in the Life — Outpatient Orthopedic

6:00 a.m.

The alarm goes off earlier than necessary, but the extra time creates a buffer before the clinic day begins. Coffee brews while emails and the schedule for the day are reviewed on a tablet at the kitchen counter. The patient load is full — post-operative knees, rotator cuff repairs, chronic low-back pain follow-ups, and a new evaluation scheduled mid-morning. A quick breakfast, a short stretch routine to loosen the lower back and shoulders, and a glance at the weather set the rhythm for the day. Before leaving, the leash is clipped onto a golden retriever named Sunny, who gets a quick walk around the neighborhood, an early-morning ritual that helps clear the mind before stepping into a fast-paced clinical environment.

6:45 a.m.

The commute is short, about twenty minutes, just enough time to mentally preview the flow of the day. Outpatient orthopedic clinics move quickly, and preparation helps reduce the sense of constant time pressure. The radio plays quietly while mentally rehearsing treatment progressions for a few complex cases scheduled later in the afternoon.

7:15 a.m.

Arriving at the clinic before the first patient provides a small but valuable advantage. Equipment is checked, resistance bands are restocked, treatment tables are cleaned, and the electronic health record system is opened to review notes from the previous sessions. One patient is approaching discharge and needs a final outcome assessment; another is not progressing as expected and may require modification to the treatment plan or consultation with the referring physician.

8:00 a.m.

The first patient arrives, a post-operative anterior cruciate ligament reconstruction. The session focuses on mobility progression, neuromuscular control, and strengthening exercises carefully advanced within surgical protocol limits. Education becomes as important as the exercises themselves — explaining why each step matters, reinforcing adherence to the home program, and managing expectations about recovery timelines. Between sets, documentation notes are entered quickly to prevent backlog later in the day.

9:30 a.m.

The morning schedule is now fully in motion. Patients rotate through treatment stations while short windows of time are used to complete charting updates. The pace requires continuous multitasking: observing movement quality, adjusting exercise difficulty, answering patient questions, and coordinating with therapy assistants who help supervise portions of treatment sessions. Each case demands attention, yet efficiency is essential to keep the schedule running smoothly.

11:00 a.m.

A new evaluation begins — a runner experiencing chronic hip pain that has limited training for several months. The assessment involves gait observation, strength testing, range-of-motion analysis, and a discussion of training habits, footwear, and recent activity changes. Developing an individualized treatment plan requires clinical reasoning (gl), but also communication skills to ensure the patient understands the recovery pathway and commits to the necessary workload outside the clinic.

12:30 p.m.

Lunch is quick and often interrupted by brief documentation catch-up. On lighter days there may be time to step outside for fresh air, but on heavier schedules the break is mostly administrative. Even so, these short pauses provide an opportunity to reset before the afternoon patient block begins.

1:00 p.m.

Afternoon sessions include a mix of progress evaluations and functional training work. One long-term patient, recovering from shoulder surgery, achieves a milestone by completing an overhead lift without compensation for the first time. Moments like this — visible, measurable functional improvement — are small but meaningful reminders of why many therapists choose the profession.

3:30 p.m.

Energy management becomes important late in the day. Maintaining consistent attention to patient safety, proper exercise technique, and accurate documentation requires sustained focus even as physical fatigue begins to build. Quick hydration breaks and short posture resets between patients help maintain stamina.

5:00 p.m.

The final patient finishes treatment, but the day is not quite over. Remaining documentation is completed, outcome measures are submitted, and the next day's schedule is reviewed to identify new evaluations or complex follow-ups that may require additional preparation.

5:45 p.m.

The commute home provides a natural transition from clinic pace to personal time. Once home, Sunny greets enthusiastically at the door, signaling the official shift away from the workday. Dinner, a short walk, and light stretching help offset the physical demands of standing and demonstrating exercises throughout the day.

10:30 p.m.

Before bed, a quick check of the next day's schedule helps set expectations, reducing early-morning decision fatigue. The routine repeats, but each day carries different clinical challenges, patient progress stories, and opportunities to refine both treatment skill and time-management efficiency — the ongoing rhythm of outpatient physical therapy practice.

SCRUB*fits*™ Reflection — Lilac Lift, DPT

"Progress in physical therapy is rarely dramatic in a single session. The work rewards clinicians who find satisfaction in small gains repeated consistently over time. If the steady rhythm of gradual improvement feels meaningful to you, this profession often becomes deeply fulfilling."

Chapter 8

Day in the Life Acute Care

5:30 a.m.

The alarm sounds early, earlier than most outpatient clinicians would ever consider, but hospital-based practice often begins before the first official patient rounds. A quick shower, coffee prepared while scanning the day's hospital census on a secure mobile app, and a light breakfast set the tone for the morning. A gray tabby cat named Milo circles the kitchen expecting breakfast first, a small but grounding ritual before stepping into a highly unpredictable clinical environment. After feeding Milo and packing a lunch, the commute begins just after 6:15 a.m., giving enough time to arrive before interdisciplinary rounds.

6:45 a.m.

Parking garages at large hospitals fill quickly, so arriving early reduces unnecessary stress. Once inside, the first stop is the therapy office to review overnight admissions, new surgical cases, and physician consults that require early mobilization assessments. Acute care schedules are rarely static; patient conditions change constantly, and flexibility is essential. The electronic record shows a mix of orthopedic surgery recoveries, cardiac patients requiring mobility evaluations, and a neurological case transferred overnight from the ICU.

7:30 a.m.

Morning interdisciplinary rounds begin. Physicians, nurses, case managers, and rehabilitation staff briefly review patient status, discharge planning needs, and mobility goals. Physical therapists play a key role in determining whether patients are safe to return home, require inpatient rehabilitation, or need skilled nursing placement. These recommendations influence both patient outcomes and hospital throughput, making clinical judgment particularly important in acute settings.

8:15 a.m.

The first evaluation involves a post-operative hip fracture patient who has been cleared for early mobilization. Vital signs are checked carefully, lines and drains are assessed, and nursing staff coordinate assistance for the initial transfer out of bed. The first standing attempt is often a major milestone for patients, requiring reassurance, safety awareness, and careful guarding techniques. Documenting tolerance to activity, assistance levels, and discharge mobility potential begins immediately after the session.

10:30 a.m.

Mid-morning brings a rapid shift in priorities. A new consult arrives for a patient recovering from cardiac surgery who must be assessed before noon discharge planning meetings. Acute care therapists constantly reprioritize schedules, balancing planned sessions with urgent referrals that impact same-day discharge decisions. Efficiency in chart review, communication with nursing staff, and quick but thorough functional assessments keeps the day moving.

12:00 p.m.

Lunch happens when possible rather than at a fixed time. Some days allow for a short break in the cafeteria; other days mean eating quickly in the therapy office while finishing documentation. Conversations with occupational therapists and case managers often continue informally over lunch, aligning discharge recommendations and coordinating patient needs across disciplines.

1:30 p.m.

Afternoon sessions include reassessments for patients who were borderline safe for discharge earlier in the day. Improvements in walking distance, stair negotiation, or transfer independence can change discharge recommendations within hours, making repeat evaluations an important part of acute care workflow. Communication with physicians and discharge planners ensures recommendations are implemented quickly so patients do not experience unnecessary delays.

3:30 p.m.

Fatigue management becomes important in the late afternoon. Acute care therapy involves frequent walking across large hospital units, repeated patient transfers, and sustained clinical concentration. Quick hydration breaks and brief posture resets between rooms help maintain physical endurance.

4:45 p.m.

The final documentation block begins, ensuring all mobility recommendations, discharge notes, and care coordination updates are complete before leaving. Acute care environments require same-day charting accuracy because discharge decisions often occur early the following morning.

5:30 p.m.

Leaving the hospital provides a noticeable shift in pace. The drive home becomes a mental decompression period, transitioning from constant clinical decision-making to personal time. At home, Milo greets at the door, dinner is prepared, and a short evening walk helps unwind after a physically active day spent across hospital floors.

10:00 p.m.

Before sleep, a quick review of the next day's starting assignments offers a preview of patient caseload complexity, allowing a smoother mental start in the morning. Acute care practice rarely offers identical days, but the constant variety of patient presentations and the opportunity to influence early recovery milestones keep the work dynamic and clinically engaging.

Chapter 9

Day in the Life
Inpatient Rehabilitation

5:45 a.m.

The alarm rings early enough to allow a calm start before a full rehabilitation day begins. Coffee brews while reviewing the day's therapy schedule on a tablet. In inpatient rehabilitation, sessions are longer and more structured than acute care or outpatient practice, so preparation helps anticipate equipment needs and therapy progression goals. Breakfast is quick but steady — oatmeal and fruit — while a beagle named Cooper waits impatiently by the door for a short morning walk before departure.

6:45 a.m.

The commute is predictable, about twenty-five minutes, giving just enough time to mentally review the patients scheduled for the morning: a stroke recovery case working toward independent transfers, a spinal cord injury patient progressing wheelchair mobility skills, and a joint replacement patient preparing for discharge home later in the week. Unlike outpatient clinics, inpatient rehabilitation often allows therapists to follow patients closely across multiple weeks, creating a strong sense of continuity in recovery progress.

7:30 a.m.

Arriving at the rehabilitation hospital, the first step is reviewing overnight nursing notes and any medical updates that might affect therapy intensity. Coordination with occupational therapists, speech-language pathologists, and nursing staff ensures each patient's daily therapy block aligns with energy levels, medication timing, and safety considerations. Interdisciplinary collaboration is constant in this setting because each therapy discipline contributes to the overall discharge readiness plan.

8:30 a.m.

The first session begins with a patient recovering from a recent stroke. Treatment focuses on gait retraining, balance work, and neuromuscular re-education designed to rebuild movement patterns affected by neurological injury. Progress can feel gradual, but small milestones — longer walking distances, improved balance reactions, more controlled transfers — represent major steps toward independence. Documentation between sessions captures functional improvements, assistance levels, and next-step therapy goals.

10:30 a.m.

The second therapy block involves a patient recovering from spinal surgery who is learning safe mobility techniques while protecting healing structures. Education plays a large role in inpatient rehabilitation, teaching patients how to move safely outside therapy sessions and preparing them for the home environment they will soon return to.

12:00 p.m.

Lunch provides a scheduled pause, often shared with the broader rehabilitation team. Informal conversations during these breaks help therapists align discharge plans, discuss patient barriers, and coordinate family training sessions needed before patients return home.

1:00 p.m.

Afternoon therapy focuses on endurance training and functional mobility progression for patients nearing discharge. Stair negotiation, car transfer simulations, and community mobility preparation become priorities as discharge dates approach. These sessions often feel particularly rewarding because functional independence improvements are clearly visible after weeks of steady work.

3:30 p.m.

Energy begins to taper slightly late in the day, but the pace remains structured. Inpatient rehabilitation schedules are predictable compared to other settings, allowing therapists to manage documentation steadily throughout the day rather than leaving large charting blocks for the evening.

4:45 p.m.

Final documentation updates are completed, progress summaries are entered, and equipment recommendations for upcoming discharges are confirmed with case management staff. Preparing these details ahead of discharge prevents delays and ensures patients transition safely to the next phase of recovery.

5:30 p.m.

The commute home offers time to mentally shift out of clinical mode. At home, Cooper greets enthusiastically, signaling the start of personal time. Dinner, a short walk, and light stretching help offset the physical demands of the day.

10:15 p.m.

Before bed, a quick glance at the next day's therapy roster helps anticipate any new admissions or discharge sessions requiring extra preparation. Inpatient rehabilitation work carries emotional investment as therapists witness long-term recovery journeys unfold, but the opportunity to see patients regain independence over weeks of consistent therapy remains one of the most fulfilling aspects of the profession.

SCRUB*fits*™ Reflection — Lilac Lift, DPT

"Many people underestimate the physical stamina required in therapy practice. Notice how the movement, lifting, positioning, and constant activity described in this chapter feel as you imagine yourself performing them daily. Physical alignment with the role matters as much as intellectual preparation."

Chapter 10

Day in the Life
Home Health

6:30 a.m.

The workday begins a little later than hospital-based roles, but preparation starts immediately. Coffee brews while reviewing the home-visit schedule on a laptop. Unlike clinic settings where patients come to the therapist, home health requires careful route planning across multiple neighborhoods to minimize drive time and maintain appointment windows. Breakfast is quick while a black Labrador named Duke waits patiently near the door, expecting his short morning walk before the first visit of the day.

7:30 a.m.

After loading therapy supplies into the car — resistance bands, portable balance tools, gait belts, and documentation tablet — the first drive begins. Travel time is a regular part of the workday in home health practice, creating natural breaks between patient visits but also requiring strong time-management skills to stay on schedule.

8:15 a.m.

The first patient is recovering from knee replacement surgery and recently discharged from inpatient rehabilitation. Entering the home environment provides a very different clinical perspective compared to hospital or outpatient settings. Narrow hallways, loose rugs, uneven flooring, and furniture placement all influence fall risk and mobility safety. Treatment focuses not only on strength and range of motion but also on practical tasks such as safe bathroom transfers, stair navigation, and strategies for moving safely within the home layout.

10:00 a.m.

The second visit involves a patient managing chronic balance deficits who has experienced multiple recent falls. Home health therapy allows clinicians to identify environmental hazards directly and recommend modifications — grab bar placement, improved lighting, removal of tripping hazards — that would be difficult to evaluate in a clinic setting. Education for both the patient and family members becomes a central component of each visit.

12:00 p.m.

Lunch is often taken in the car between visits, providing a brief administrative window to complete documentation while parked safely. Many home health therapists complete notes immediately after each visit to avoid large documentation backlogs later in the day.

1:30 p.m.

Afternoon visits may include reassessments or discharge planning sessions. One patient nearing independence practices community mobility tasks, such as safely entering and exiting a vehicle, while another focuses on endurance training to improve tolerance for daily household activities. The variety of living environments keeps clinical decision-making dynamic, as each home presents different mobility challenges.

3:30 p.m.

The final visit of the day involves caregiver training, teaching a family member safe transfer techniques to reduce injury risk for both the patient and caregiver. These sessions often extend slightly longer than planned because confidence-building and hands-on practice are essential before therapy services conclude.

4:45 p.m.

Driving home marks the administrative wrap-up period. Final documentation entries are completed through secure mobile systems, and the next day's visit confirmations are reviewed. Because travel is built into the schedule, many therapists find the day feels less rushed than clinic-based roles, though time-management discipline remains essential.

5:30 p.m.

Back at home, Duke greets enthusiastically, ready for his evening walk. The workday ends without the noise of a busy clinic, replaced by the quieter rhythm that often characterizes home health practice. Dinner, light stretching, and personal time help transition fully out of work mode.

10:30 p.m.

A final glance at tomorrow's travel route ensures appointment timing is realistic. Home health therapy combines clinical care with mobility across communities, offering independence and scheduling flexibility for therapists who enjoy variety, autonomy, and direct insight into how patients function within their real-world environments.

Chapter 11

Day in the Life Skilled Nursing Facility

6:00 a.m.

The day begins early, but unlike hospital-based roles, the pace of the morning feels more predictable. Coffee brews while reviewing the patient list for the day — a mix of short-term rehabilitation residents recovering from surgeries and long-term residents working on mobility maintenance programs. Breakfast is quick while a small terrier named Penny circles the kitchen, anticipating her morning walk before departure.

6:45 a.m.

The commute is short, allowing arrival before most therapy sessions begin. Skilled nursing facilities often operate on tightly coordinated therapy schedules that must align with medication timing, nursing care routines, and meal schedules. Checking overnight nursing notes and medical updates is the first step to identify any residents who may need modified therapy intensity due to changes in medical status.

7:30 a.m.

Morning therapy sessions begin with residents who prefer earlier treatment times. The first session focuses on transfer training for a resident recovering from hip surgery, emphasizing safe sit-to-stand mechanics and walker use. Many sessions in this setting involve functional mobility training tied directly to daily living activities — moving from bed to chair, navigating hallways, and safely managing bathroom transfers.

9:30 a.m.

The next resident is working on balance and fall-prevention strategies. Skilled nursing therapy often includes repetition-based functional training, reinforcing safe movement patterns that residents must use consistently outside therapy sessions. Communication with nursing staff ensures that recommended mobility assistance levels are followed throughout the day.

11:30 a.m.

Documentation is completed between sessions whenever possible. Skilled nursing environments require detailed recording of treatment minutes, functional progress, and discharge planning indicators tied to reimbursement and regulatory requirements. Efficient charting habits help prevent late-day administrative overload.

12:30 p.m.

Lunch offers a brief pause, often spent in the staff breakroom exchanging updates with occupational therapists and nursing personnel about residents approaching discharge readiness. Coordinated discharge planning is essential to ensure patients transition safely back home or to lower levels of care.

1:30 p.m.

Afternoon sessions include gait training in longer facility hallways, endurance walking programs, and stair training for residents preparing to return home. Family education sessions sometimes occur during these hours, allowing caregivers to learn safe transfer techniques and mobility assistance strategies before discharge.

3:30 p.m.

Energy management becomes important late in the day. Skilled nursing therapy often involves frequent standing, guarding residents during walking practice, and repeated transfer assistance. Brief hydration breaks and posture resets help maintain stamina through the final sessions.

4:45 p.m.

Final documentation is completed, therapy minutes are verified, and the next day's treatment schedule is reviewed. Because regulatory documentation accuracy is closely monitored in this setting, ensuring chart completion before departure reduces the need for after-hours administrative work.

5:30 p.m.

The commute home signals the shift from clinical pace to personal time. Penny greets enthusiastically at the door, ready for her evening walk. Dinner, light stretching, and relaxation help offset the physical demands of assisting residents throughout the day.

10:15 p.m.

Before bed, a quick review of the next day's patient assignments provides a preview of therapy priorities. Skilled nursing practice offers the opportunity to support both short-term recovery and long-term mobility preservation, creating a steady rhythm of care focused on maintaining independence and preventing functional decline among aging populations.

SCRUB*fits*™ Reflection — Lilac Lift, DPT

"Motivation is one of the most important therapeutic tools a physical therapist carries. If encouraging patients through difficult recoveries energizes you, the work often feels purposeful. If repeated motivational effort feels draining, that signal deserves attention."

Chapter 12

Day in the Life Pediatric Outpatient

6:15 a.m.

The morning begins early, not because the clinic opens particularly early, but because preparation helps create a calmer pace for a day that requires constant energy and engagement. Coffee brews while reviewing the pediatric therapy schedule, which includes a mix of developmental delay cases, post-surgical orthopedic follow-ups, and children working on balance and coordination goals. Breakfast is quick while a small orange tabby cat named Luna winds around the kitchen chair waiting for breakfast before the commute begins.

7:15 a.m.

The drive to the clinic takes about twenty minutes, providing time to mentally preview treatment ideas for the day. Pediatric therapy sessions require creativity and flexibility, as treatment activities are often delivered through play-based interventions designed to keep children engaged while targeting functional goals.

7:45 a.m.

Arriving early allows time to prepare therapy stations — mats, balance equipment, stepping platforms, and coordination tools are set up before the first patient arrives. Pediatric clinics often rely heavily on visual engagement, so arranging equipment strategically helps sessions flow smoothly without frequent interruptions.

8:30 a.m.

The first session begins with a young child working on gross motor development. Activities include obstacle navigation, balance stepping exercises, and movement games designed to strengthen coordination while maintaining engagement. Encouragement and pacing are essential, as young patients often respond best when therapy feels playful rather than structured.

10:00 a.m.

The next appointment involves a school-age child recovering from orthopedic surgery. Treatment focuses on range-of-motion progression and strengthening exercises delivered through interactive tasks that maintain attention. Communication with parents becomes a key component of the session, reinforcing home exercise participation and explaining recovery milestones.

12:00 p.m.

Lunch offers a brief break and an opportunity to complete documentation. Pediatric therapists often document progress notes immediately after sessions to maintain accuracy while details remain fresh.

1:00 p.m.

Afternoon sessions include coordination training for children with developmental motor challenges. Treatment involves repetition, patience, and careful progression, often celebrating small improvements that represent meaningful functional gains over time.

3:30 p.m.

Energy management becomes important late in the day, particularly when sessions require constant movement, demonstration, and engagement. Hydration breaks between appointments help maintain stamina while preparing for the final sessions.

4:45 p.m.

The last patient finishes, equipment is reset, and final documentation is completed. Reviewing the next day's schedule helps anticipate any new evaluations that may require additional preparation.

5:30 p.m.

The commute home marks the transition out of the clinic environment. At home, Luna greets at the door, signaling the shift to personal time. Dinner, relaxation, and light stretching help offset the physical demands of demonstrating activities throughout the day.

10:30 p.m.

Before sleep, a brief review of tomorrow's appointments provides a mental preview of upcoming sessions. Pediatric outpatient therapy requires sustained energy and creativity, but the opportunity to support developmental progress and long-term functional independence offers a uniquely rewarding rhythm to the workday.

Chapter 13

Day in the Life Sports Performance Clinic

6:00 a.m.

The alarm sounds early because many athletes prefer training sessions before school or work hours. Coffee brews while reviewing the day's appointment list — post-operative ACL rehabilitation cases, shoulder stability work for overhead athletes, and return-to-sport progression sessions for individuals nearing clearance. Breakfast is quick while a border collie named Jax waits by the door for a short morning walk before departure.

6:45 a.m.

The commute is brief, and arriving early allows time to prepare the performance space. Resistance equipment is arranged, agility ladders are set out, and testing tools used for strength and functional performance assessments are calibrated before the first athlete arrives.

7:30 a.m.

The first session involves a collegiate athlete progressing through late-stage knee rehabilitation. Treatment focuses on controlled plyometric drills, movement pattern correction, and strength testing to measure readiness for higher-level activity. Communication emphasizes both performance goals and injury prevention strategies, ensuring progression remains safe and measurable.

9:00 a.m.

Mid-morning sessions include shoulder rehabilitation for a baseball pitcher recovering from overuse injury. Treatment integrates mobility restoration, rotator cuff strengthening, and progressive throwing mechanics work coordinated with the athlete's training staff. Collaboration with coaches and athletic trainers is a routine part of this environment.

11:30 a.m.

Documentation is completed between sessions while reviewing performance metrics recorded during testing activities. Tracking measurable outcomes helps guide safe return-to-play decisions.

12:30 p.m.

Lunch provides a short reset before the afternoon training block begins. Many sports clinics operate on staggered schedules, allowing athletes to attend sessions around school or practice times.

1:30 p.m.

Afternoon appointments include general fitness clients recovering from orthopedic injuries who are transitioning back into exercise routines. Sessions blend rehabilitation principles with performance training, helping individuals rebuild strength while minimizing reinjury risk.

3:30 p.m.

Energy management becomes important as later sessions often involve high-intensity movement demonstrations and coaching. Hydration and quick stretching between sessions help maintain physical endurance throughout the day.

5:30 p.m.

The final athlete finishes training, equipment is reset, and performance data is entered into tracking systems. Reviewing the next day's athlete roster helps anticipate equipment setup and progression planning.

6:15 p.m.

The commute home provides a shift from coaching-focused energy to personal time. At home, Jax greets enthusiastically, ready for an evening walk. Dinner and relaxation help transition away from the high-energy clinic environment.

10:30 p.m.

A quick review of the next day's schedule ensures readiness for early athlete sessions. Sports performance practice blends rehabilitation science with athletic performance coaching, creating a dynamic environment where therapists work closely with motivated individuals striving to return to peak physical ability.

SCRUB*fits*™ Reflection — Lilac Lift, DPT

"Therapy schedules can be tightly paced, with productivity expectations shaping how each hour is structured. Some clinicians enjoy this steady operational rhythm, while others prefer more flexible workflows. Long-term satisfaction often depends on how well that pace fits your working style."

Chapter 14

Day in the Life Neurological Rehabilitation

5:45 a.m.

The morning begins quietly, with coffee brewing while reviewing the therapy caseload for the day. Neurological rehabilitation schedules often include patients recovering from stroke, traumatic brain injury, Parkinson's disease, and spinal cord injury (gl), each requiring individualized treatment pacing and preparation. Breakfast is simple while a rescue mixed-breed dog named Bailey waits patiently for a short morning walk before the commute begins.

6:45 a.m.

The drive to the rehabilitation center takes about twenty minutes, providing time to mentally review treatment goals for patients scheduled in the morning block. Neurological rehabilitation requires careful attention to fatigue levels, cognitive engagement, and movement pattern retraining, so planning session flow ahead of time helps maximize therapeutic benefit.

7:30 a.m.

Arriving early allows time to review overnight updates from nursing staff and confirm any medical status changes that could affect therapy intensity. Coordination with occupational therapists and speech-language pathologists ensures interdisciplinary treatment goals remain aligned.

8:30 a.m.

The first session focuses on a patient recovering from stroke, working on gait retraining using body-weight-supported treadmill systems. Sessions often move at a slower pace than orthopedic settings, emphasizing repetition, motor learning principles, and safety monitoring. Small improvements in coordination or balance represent meaningful progress, even when changes appear subtle.

10:30 a.m.

The next patient session involves balance and postural control training for an individual with Parkinson's disease. Treatment incorporates cueing strategies, functional movement repetition, and caregiver education to reinforce safe mobility practices outside therapy sessions.

12:00 p.m.

Lunch provides a scheduled pause, often shared with the rehabilitation team. Informal discussions during this time help coordinate discharge timelines and long-term therapy planning.

1:00 p.m.

Afternoon therapy sessions focus on endurance building and functional mobility training for patients progressing toward discharge readiness. Teaching adaptive movement strategies becomes a key component, helping patients and families develop confidence in daily activities.

3:30 p.m.

Late-day sessions require sustained attention to both physical assistance and patient motivation, as neurological recovery can involve gradual, incremental progress. Hydration breaks and short posture resets between patients help maintain stamina.

4:45 p.m.

Final documentation is completed, noting functional gains, assistance levels, and recommendations for the following therapy sessions. Accurate charting is essential for continuity across interdisciplinary care teams.

5:30 p.m.

The commute home marks the transition out of the clinical environment. Bailey greets enthusiastically at the door, ready for an evening walk. Dinner, stretching, and quiet time help offset the physical demands of assisting patients throughout the day.

10:15 p.m.

Before sleep, reviewing the next day's therapy assignments provides a preview of patient progression needs. Neurological rehabilitation work requires patience, sustained focus, and careful progression planning, but the opportunity to help patients regain functional independence following life-altering conditions remains one of the most meaningful aspects of the profession.

Chapter 15

Day in the Life Rural Community Hospital

5:30 a.m.

The morning begins early, typical for hospital-based roles, but rural settings often require additional flexibility because therapists may cover multiple patient populations in the same day. Coffee brews while reviewing the therapy caseload remotely, which includes orthopedic post-surgical patients, a medical admission requiring mobility assessment, and an outpatient follow-up visit scheduled later in the afternoon. Breakfast is quick while a small Australian shepherd named Scout waits by the door for a short morning walk before the commute begins.

6:30 a.m.

The drive to the hospital takes about thirty minutes through quieter country roads, providing time to mentally prepare for the day's varied responsibilities. Rural practice often requires therapists to function as generalists, moving between inpatient, outpatient, and emergency consult roles depending on daily needs.

7:15 a.m.

Arriving at the hospital, the first step is checking overnight admissions and reviewing any therapy consults placed by physicians. Communication with nursing staff helps identify patients who may require early mobility evaluations or discharge readiness assessments.

8:00 a.m.

The first session involves a post-operative knee replacement patient preparing for discharge the following day. Treatment focuses on walking tolerance, stair practice, and safe transfer techniques, ensuring the patient meets discharge mobility benchmarks before leaving the hospital.

10:00 a.m.

A call comes from the medical unit requesting a mobility evaluation for a patient admitted overnight with respiratory complications. Acute mobility assessments require quick clinical judgment to determine safe activity levels while coordinating closely with nursing staff to monitor vital signs and patient tolerance.

12:00 p.m.

Lunch is taken in the staff breakroom while completing documentation from the morning sessions. In smaller hospitals, therapists often complete charting steadily throughout the day to maintain workflow efficiency.

1:00 p.m.

Afternoon responsibilities shift to outpatient therapy visits conducted within the hospital's rehabilitation department. One patient recovering from shoulder surgery works through strengthening progression exercises while another attends a follow-up mobility session after discharge from inpatient care.

3:30 p.m.

Late-afternoon responsibilities include reassessing a patient whose discharge depends on mobility improvement following morning therapy. Coordinating with physicians and case management ensures discharge decisions are made efficiently when mobility benchmarks are achieved.

4:45 p.m.

Final documentation is completed, therapy equipment is organized, and the next day's mixed caseload is reviewed. Rural practice often requires rapid adjustment between care settings, making organization and adaptability essential skills.

5:30 p.m.

The drive home provides a quiet transition from the day's varied responsibilities. At home, Scout greets enthusiastically, ready for an evening walk before dinner and relaxation.

10:15 p.m.

Before bed, a quick look at the next day's schedule helps anticipate any cross-setting responsibilities that may arise. Rural community hospital practice offers wide clinical variety and strong community relationships, creating a dynamic workday shaped by flexibility and broad clinical skill use.

Chapter 16

Day in the Life Travel Physical Therapist

6:30 a.m.

The morning routine varies depending on the assignment location, but flexibility is a constant feature of travel practice. Coffee brews in a temporary apartment kitchen while reviewing the clinic schedule for the day. Travel therapists often accept contracts in high-demand regions, meaning patient volumes can be busy from the start. Breakfast is quick while a video call home provides a brief connection before the workday begins, helping maintain personal routines even while working in a new city.

7:30 a.m.

The commute to the contracted facility may be unfamiliar during the first few weeks of an assignment, so leaving early helps account for traffic patterns still being learned. Many travel therapists use navigation apps consistently until local routes become second nature.

8:00 a.m.

Arriving at the clinic, the first task is reviewing patient charts and confirming documentation expectations specific to the facility. Each assignment introduces new electronic record systems, workflow processes, and scheduling structures, requiring adaptability and quick learning during the initial days of a contract.

9:00 a.m.

The first patient session involves post-operative rehabilitation for a knee replacement patient progressing through strengthening and mobility milestones. Travel therapists must quickly integrate into the clinic team while maintaining the same clinical standards expected of permanent staff, often balancing patient care with the ongoing process of learning facility-specific procedures.

11:30 a.m.

Midday documentation is completed between sessions to stay current with facility expectations. Many travel therapists prioritize real-time charting to avoid administrative work accumulating after clinic hours.

12:30 p.m.

Lunch may be taken with clinic staff, providing an opportunity to build rapport with colleagues and learn informal workflow tips that help assignments run smoothly.

1:30 p.m.

Afternoon sessions include reassessments and patient education visits. Because travel therapists frequently enter clinics experiencing staffing shortages, caseloads can be full, requiring efficient time management and strong clinical organization.

4:45 p.m.

End-of-day documentation is finalized, and the next day's patient schedule is reviewed. Travel therapists often double-check appointment expectations early in assignments to ensure smooth transitions across unfamiliar systems.

5:30 p.m.

After leaving the clinic, the evening may include exploring the new city, exercising, or connecting with friends and family remotely. Travel assignments often provide opportunities to experience different regions while maintaining clinical practice.

10:30 p.m.

Before sleep, reviewing the next day's clinic schedule helps anticipate any new evaluations or complex cases. Travel physical therapy offers variety, geographic flexibility, and exposure to diverse clinical environments, but it also requires adaptability, strong organization, and comfort working within constantly changing workplace systems.

Chapter 17

Day in the Life Academic Medical Center

5:15 a.m.

The day begins early, reflecting the complexity and pace often associated with large academic hospitals. Coffee brews while reviewing the patient caseload, which includes complex post-surgical cases, neurological recovery patients, and consults from specialty medical teams. Breakfast is quick while a Maine Coon cat named Atlas watches from the kitchen counter, expecting breakfast before the morning commute begins.

6:15 a.m.

The drive into the city requires a bit more planning due to traffic patterns around major medical campuses. Many clinicians arrive early to secure parking and allow time to review overnight clinical updates before formal rounds begin.

7:00 a.m.

Upon arrival, the first task is reviewing electronic medical records for overnight changes in patient condition, surgical updates, or new therapy consults placed by attending physicians. Academic centers frequently manage high-acuity patients, requiring careful attention to medical complexity before beginning mobility sessions.

7:45 a.m.

Interdisciplinary rounds begin with physicians, residents, nurses, case managers, and therapy staff discussing patient status and discharge planning. Physical therapists play a central role in determining mobility readiness, rehabilitation needs, and projected discharge pathways for patients transitioning to inpatient rehabilitation, home health, or outpatient care.

9:00 a.m.

The first session involves early mobilization for a patient recovering from complex spinal surgery. Coordination with nursing staff ensures monitoring equipment is safely managed while initiating assisted standing and walking activities. Careful guarding and close vital sign monitoring are essential due to the patient's medical status.

11:00 a.m.

Mid-morning sessions often involve patients with multiple comorbidities requiring cautious progression. Clinical decision-making includes balancing mobility benefits with patient tolerance, fatigue, and safety considerations.

12:30 p.m.

Lunch offers a short break, often spent informally discussing complex cases with colleagues or reviewing research updates relevant to specialty rehabilitation protocols commonly implemented in academic settings.

1:30 p.m.

Afternoon responsibilities may include mentoring physical therapy students completing clinical rotations. Teaching moments occur throughout patient sessions, guiding students through evaluation techniques, clinical reasoning, and documentation standards.

3:30 p.m.

Late-day sessions include reassessments for patients approaching discharge readiness. Recommendations are communicated directly to case management and medical teams to support coordinated discharge planning.

4:45 p.m.

Final documentation is completed, and new consult requests for the following day are reviewed. Academic centers often require timely charting to maintain communication across large interdisciplinary teams.

5:30 p.m.

Leaving the hospital signals a transition from the fast-paced clinical environment to personal time. At home, Atlas greets at the door, marking the shift away from the workday. Dinner, relaxation, and light stretching help offset the physical demands of assisting patients throughout the day.

10:00 p.m.

Before sleep, reviewing the next day's assignment list helps anticipate complex patient needs. Practice in an academic medical center offers exposure to advanced clinical cases, teaching opportunities, and interdisciplinary collaboration that continually expands clinical skill and professional growth.

Chapter 18

Day in the Life Early Intervention (Birth to Three)

6:30 a.m.

The morning begins at a steady pace, typical for community-based pediatric work. Coffee brews while reviewing the day's visit schedule, which includes several early-intervention home visits for infants and toddlers working on developmental mobility milestones. Breakfast is quick while a miniature dachshund named Pepper circles the kitchen, ready for a short morning walk before the commute begins.

7:30 a.m.

Therapy materials are packed into a rolling bag — soft mats, developmental toys, positioning supports, and educational handouts for parents. Early intervention practice often takes place in homes or childcare settings, so preparation focuses on portable equipment that supports developmental play-based therapy.

8:30 a.m.

The first visit involves an infant working on head control and early rolling milestones. Therapy sessions emphasize parent coaching, demonstrating positioning techniques and guided movement activities that caregivers can safely practice throughout the week. Family education forms a central component of early-intervention therapy because progress depends heavily on consistent practice outside formal sessions.

10:00 a.m.

The second home visit focuses on a toddler working on early walking skills. Treatment includes balance activities, supported standing transitions, and play-based stepping exercises designed to build strength while maintaining engagement. Observing how the child moves within the natural home environment provides valuable insight into real-world developmental challenges.

12:00 p.m.

Lunch is often taken between visits, sometimes in the car while completing brief documentation notes. Completing charting immediately after each session helps maintain accuracy and reduces administrative workload later in the day.

1:30 p.m.

Afternoon sessions include consultation with parents of a child receiving services for developmental delay. Discussions focus on home routines, safe play activities, and strategies to incorporate therapeutic movement practice into daily family life. Collaboration with speech and occupational therapists is common to ensure developmental goals remain coordinated across disciplines.

3:30 p.m.

The final visit of the day involves reassessment of developmental milestones for a child approaching transition into preschool-based services. Documentation includes functional progress updates, goal revisions, and coordination with the broader early-intervention team.

4:45 p.m.

After the final visit, documentation is completed through secure mobile systems, and the next day's travel route is reviewed. Community-based pediatric practice requires careful scheduling to maintain realistic travel time between appointments.

5:30 p.m.

Returning home marks the transition to personal time. Pepper greets enthusiastically, ready for an evening walk. Dinner, relaxation, and light stretching help unwind after a day spent traveling between home visits.

10:15 p.m.

Before sleep, reviewing the next day's schedule helps anticipate developmental focus areas for upcoming sessions. Early-intervention physical therapy centers on guiding families as much as treating children, creating a workday built around coaching, developmental progress monitoring, and supporting early mobility independence during the most formative years of growth.

SCRUB*fits*™ Reflection — Lilac Lift, DPT

"Recovery journeys often include setbacks. Therapists who remain patient and solution-focused during slow progress tend to thrive in this field. Consider how you typically respond when improvement takes longer than expected — your natural response is an important alignment indicator."

Chapter 19

Day in the Life Industrial / Workplace Rehabilitation

6:00 a.m.

The day begins early because many industrial rehabilitation clinics align their schedules with manufacturing and warehouse shift patterns. Coffee brews while reviewing the patient list for the day, which includes workers recovering from lifting injuries, repetitive strain conditions, and post-surgical orthopedic recoveries preparing to return to physically demanding jobs. Breakfast is quick while a husky named Nova waits by the door for a short walk before departure.

6:45 a.m.

The commute is brief, and arriving early allows time to prepare functional work-simulation equipment used during therapy sessions. Industrial rehabilitation often includes lifting stations, pushing and pulling resistance devices, and work-simulation tasks designed to mirror the physical demands of specific occupations.

7:30 a.m.

The first session begins with a worker recovering from a shoulder injury who is progressing through return-to-work conditioning. Treatment focuses on graded strengthening tasks that simulate workplace movements while monitoring technique and fatigue levels to ensure safe progression.

9:00 a.m.

Mid-morning sessions include ergonomic education for employees returning to repetitive task environments. Teaching proper lifting mechanics, workstation setup adjustments, and injury-prevention strategies becomes a major component of this practice setting.

11:30 a.m.

Documentation is completed between sessions, often including functional capacity assessment updates used by employers, case managers, and insurance representatives to determine readiness for modified or full-duty return to work.

12:30 p.m.

Lunch provides a brief administrative reset while reviewing the afternoon caseload. Some clinics hold short interdisciplinary meetings with occupational health teams to discuss worker progress and anticipated return-to-work timelines.

1:30 p.m.

Afternoon sessions involve structured conditioning programs designed to rebuild endurance and physical tolerance for job-specific demands. Workers may perform simulated lifting sequences, climbing activities, or repetitive task drills that mirror real occupational responsibilities.

3:30 p.m.

Energy management becomes important later in the day as sessions often involve demonstration of high-effort functional tasks. Hydration breaks and short posture resets help maintain stamina through the final patient visits.

4:45 p.m.

Final documentation includes functional progress summaries and updated work-restriction recommendations communicated to case managers and occupational health coordinators.

5:30 p.m.

Leaving the clinic signals the shift back to personal time. At home, Nova greets enthusiastically, ready for an evening run. Dinner, stretching, and relaxation help offset the physical demands of demonstrating job-simulation tasks throughout the day.

10:15 p.m.

Before bed, reviewing the next day's schedule helps anticipate any new functional capacity evaluations requiring extended testing time. Industrial rehabilitation practice blends clinical care with occupational performance training, focusing on restoring safe work capacity while reducing the risk of reinjury for individuals returning to physically demanding occupations.

Chapter 20
Day in the Life Telehealth Rehabilitation

7:00 a.m.

The workday begins slightly later than many in-person clinical settings, but preparation still starts early. Coffee brews while logging into the secure telehealth platform to review the day's virtual appointment schedule. Sessions include post-surgical mobility follow-ups, chronic pain management visits, and exercise-progression check-ins for patients living in remote areas. Breakfast is quick while a Siamese cat named Willow stretches across the keyboard, demanding attention before the first session begins.

7:45 a.m.

The home office setup is checked carefully — camera positioning, lighting, and resistance bands arranged nearby for demonstration. Telehealth sessions rely heavily on clear visual communication, so small technical adjustments can make a significant difference in patient engagement and safety.

8:00 a.m.

The first virtual appointment begins with a patient recovering from knee surgery. The session includes guided range-of-motion exercises, observation of walking mechanics through the patient's camera setup, and adjustments to the home exercise program based on observed movement patterns. Education becomes a central component of telehealth care, as patients must often perform exercises independently between visits.

9:30 a.m.

The next session focuses on chronic low-back pain management. Treatment emphasizes posture correction, ergonomic coaching for home workstations, and guided strengthening exercises using household equipment when formal therapy tools are not available.

11:30 a.m.

Documentation is completed between sessions, allowing real-time entry of exercise progressions and patient feedback. Telehealth workflows often make charting more immediate because clinicians transition directly between sessions without travel time.

12:30 p.m.

Lunch offers a short break away from the screen. A brief walk outside helps reset before the afternoon appointment block begins.

1:30 p.m.

Afternoon visits include reassessment sessions for patients nearing discharge from therapy. Functional progress is evaluated through guided movement testing performed within the patient's home environment, offering direct insight into daily mobility challenges.

3:30 p.m.

Energy management becomes important late in the day, particularly with extended screen time. Short stretching breaks and hydration help maintain focus through the final sessions.

4:45 p.m.

The final documentation block is completed, and the next day's appointment schedule is reviewed. Telehealth practice often allows flexible scheduling, but preparation remains essential to ensure each patient has the necessary equipment and setup for effective sessions.

5:15 p.m.

Logging out of the platform signals the end of the clinical day without the traditional commute. At home, Willow returns for attention, marking the transition into personal time. Dinner, relaxation, and light stretching help close the day.

10:30 p.m.

Before sleep, reviewing the next day's caseload helps anticipate any new evaluation sessions that may require additional preparation. Telehealth rehabilitation offers flexibility and expanded patient access to care, particularly for individuals in remote locations, while still requiring careful communication, patient education, and strong clinical observation skills to deliver effective treatment at a distance.

SCRUB*fits*™ Reflection — Lilac Lift, DPT

"Physical therapy blends clinical science with human connection. For many clinicians, the ongoing relationships built with patients become one of the most meaningful parts of the profession. Notice whether continuity of care feels energizing or emotionally heavy for you over time."

Chapter 21

Day in the Life Military Rehabilitation

5:00 a.m.

The alarm rings early, matching the rhythm of many military installations where physical training and operational schedules begin before sunrise. Coffee brews while reviewing the day's rehabilitation schedule, which includes service members recovering from orthopedic injuries, conditioning programs for return-to-duty readiness, and follow-up mobility assessments. Breakfast is quick while a German shepherd named Ranger waits by the door for a brief morning walk before departure.

5:45 a.m.

The commute onto the base requires additional time for security entry procedures, so leaving early helps avoid delays. Once inside the rehabilitation facility, the first step is reviewing updated medical notes and duty-status changes that may affect therapy intensity.

6:30 a.m.

Morning sessions often begin earlier than civilian clinics to align with unit schedules. The first appointment involves a service member progressing through knee rehabilitation following ligament reconstruction. Treatment includes strength progression, agility drills, and movement retraining designed to restore performance capacity required for duty responsibilities.

8:30 a.m.

The next session focuses on shoulder rehabilitation for a service member recovering from repetitive training injury. Education includes injury-prevention strategies and conditioning techniques that can be incorporated into regular physical training routines.

10:30 a.m.

Documentation is completed between sessions, including updates to functional readiness assessments used to determine return-to-duty status. Collaboration with physicians and command medical personnel ensures rehabilitation progress aligns with operational requirements.

12:00 p.m.

Lunch provides a short break and an opportunity to coordinate with athletic trainers and strength-conditioning staff supporting service member readiness programs.

1:00 p.m.

Afternoon sessions involve conditioning circuits designed to rebuild endurance and mobility for individuals nearing full-duty clearance. Functional testing may include load-carry simulations, obstacle navigation drills, and endurance mobility tasks that mirror operational activities.

3:30 p.m.

Late-day sessions often include reassessments for service members approaching discharge from rehabilitation programs. Communication of readiness levels is documented carefully, as these recommendations influence duty assignment decisions.

4:45 p.m.

Final documentation is completed, the next day's therapy roster is reviewed, and equipment used for functional training sessions is reset for the following morning.

5:30 p.m.

Leaving the base marks the transition from the structured clinical environment to personal time. At home, Ranger greets enthusiastically, ready for an evening walk. Dinner and relaxation help offset the physical demands of demonstrating performance-based rehabilitation tasks throughout the day.

10:00 p.m.

Before sleep, reviewing the next day's schedule helps anticipate upcoming evaluations and return-to-duty testing sessions. Military rehabilitation practice combines clinical care with performance readiness, creating a work environment focused on restoring strength, resilience, and operational mobility for service members returning to active roles.

Chapter 22

Day in the Life Pain Management Rehabilitation

6:15 a.m.

The day begins with a slower start compared to hospital settings, but preparation remains important. Coffee brews while reviewing the schedule, which includes patients managing chronic musculoskeletal pain, post-surgical recovery cases experiencing prolonged discomfort, and individuals participating in multidisciplinary rehabilitation programs. Breakfast is quick while a calico cat named Ember circles the kitchen before settling near the window as the commute begins.

7:15 a.m.

Arriving at the clinic early allows time to review patient histories and identify any medication or treatment updates documented by physicians or behavioral health specialists. Pain management rehabilitation often involves interdisciplinary collaboration, requiring awareness of psychological, pharmacological, and functional treatment components.

8:00 a.m.

The first session involves a patient with chronic low-back pain working on graded movement exposure techniques designed to rebuild tolerance for daily activity. Education plays a major role in these sessions, helping patients understand the difference between safe discomfort associated with recovery and warning signs that require caution.

9:30 a.m.

The next appointment focuses on a patient recovering from shoulder surgery who has developed prolonged movement avoidance due to fear of reinjury. Treatment integrates gentle mobility progression, pacing strategies, and confidence-building exercises that gradually restore functional movement.

11:30 a.m.

Documentation is completed between sessions, capturing functional progress and patient-reported outcome measures used to track long-term rehabilitation success.

12:30 p.m.

Lunch provides a short pause and an opportunity to coordinate briefly with behavioral health colleagues involved in the multidisciplinary program, aligning treatment strategies for patients receiving integrated care.

1:30 p.m.

Afternoon sessions include functional activity training for individuals preparing to return to work following extended recovery periods. Treatment emphasizes endurance building, pacing strategies, and sustainable activity progression to prevent flare-ups.

3:30 p.m.

Late-day sessions often involve reassessments of functional progress and updates to long-term rehabilitation plans. Maintaining patient motivation is a key component of pain management practice, as progress may occur gradually over extended timelines.

4:45 p.m.

Final documentation is completed, outcome tracking forms are updated, and the next day's patient schedule is reviewed.

5:30 p.m.

Returning home signals the transition into personal time. Ember greets at the door, marking the end of the clinical day. Dinner, stretching, and relaxation help offset the physical demands of demonstrating exercises throughout the day.

10:15 p.m.

Before sleep, reviewing the next day's schedule provides a preview of patient progression needs. Pain management rehabilitation requires patience, communication skill, and long-term clinical planning, creating a practice environment centered on helping individuals rebuild movement confidence and sustainable activity levels over time.

SCRUB*fits*™ Reflection — Lilac Lift, DPT

"The most sustainable therapy careers are built not only on clinical skill, but on pacing — learning how to deliver high-

quality care while protecting your own physical and mental endurance. Alignment in this profession often reveals itself in how sustainable the daily rhythm feels across months and years."

Chapter 23

The 101 — Top 101 Questions About Becoming a Physical Therapist

1. What does a physical therapist actually do on a daily basis?

Physical therapists evaluate movement limitations, design treatment plans to restore mobility and function, and guide patients through exercises and functional activities intended to reduce pain, improve strength, and support recovery after injury, surgery, or illness. While this description sounds straightforward, the daily experience of the role varies significantly depending on the clinical setting. In outpatient clinics, therapists often manage tightly scheduled patient sessions throughout the day, moving quickly between evaluations, treatment progressions, and documentation. In hospitals or rehabilitation centers, the pace may be influenced by medical complexity, interdisciplinary rounds, and discharge planning timelines. In home health settings, travel between patient homes becomes part of the daily workflow, while academic or specialty centers may include teaching, research, or advanced clinical case management responsibilities.

Beyond hands-on treatment, a substantial portion of the job involves clinical decision-making. Therapists continuously assess whether patients are progressing appropriately, determine when treatment plans should be modified, and communicate recommendations to physicians, case managers, and other healthcare professionals involved in the patient's care. Documentation is another consistent component of daily work, as therapists must record treatment interventions, patient responses, and functional progress in compliance with regulatory and reimbursement requirements. These administrative responsibilities, while often less visible to students exploring the profession, play a significant role in shaping the rhythm of the workday.

Equally important is the educational aspect of the role. Physical therapists spend considerable time teaching patients how to perform exercises safely, explaining injury recovery timelines, and coaching individuals on movement strategies that reduce reinjury risk. Much of a patient's long-term improvement depends on what happens outside the clinic, making patient education and adherence coaching essential professional skills.

Although the profession is widely associated with exercise-based treatment, the role also requires strong interpersonal communication, time-management ability, and physical stamina. Therapists often spend long periods standing, demonstrating exercises, assisting with mobility tasks, and maintaining attention across multiple patient cases simultaneously. Over time, the daily responsibilities combine clinical expertise, physical activity, problem-solving, and patient coaching into a role that is both intellectually engaging and physically demanding.

Ultimately, what a physical therapist does each day depends heavily on the environment in which they practice, but the central purpose remains consistent: helping individuals regain movement, restore independence, and return to meaningful daily activities through evidence-based rehabilitation care.

1. What does a physical therapist actually do on a daily basis?

Physical therapists evaluate movement limitations, design treatment plans to restore mobility and function, and guide patients through exercises and functional activities intended to reduce pain, improve strength, and support recovery after injury, surgery, or illness. While this description sounds straightforward, the daily experience of the role varies significantly depending on the clinical setting. In outpatient clinics, therapists often manage tightly scheduled patient sessions throughout the day, moving quickly between evaluations, treatment progressions, and documentation. In hospitals or rehabilitation centers, the pace may be influenced by medical complexity, interdisciplinary rounds, and discharge planning timelines. In home health settings, travel between patient homes becomes part of the daily workflow, while academic or specialty centers may include teaching, research, or advanced clinical case management responsibilities.

Beyond hands-on treatment, a substantial portion of the job involves clinical decision-making. Therapists continuously assess whether patients are progressing appropriately, determine when treatment plans should be modified, and communicate recommendations to physicians, case managers, and other healthcare professionals involved in the patient's care. Documentation is another consistent component of daily work, as therapists must record treatment interventions, patient responses, and functional progress in compliance with regulatory and reimbursement requirements. These administrative responsibilities, while often less visible to students exploring the profession, play a significant role in shaping the rhythm of the workday.

Equally important is the educational aspect of the role. Physical therapists spend considerable time teaching patients how to perform exercises safely, explaining injury recovery timelines, and coaching individuals on movement strategies that reduce reinjury risk. Much of a patient's long-term improvement depends on what happens outside the clinic, making patient education and adherence coaching essential professional skills.

Although the profession is widely associated with exercise-based treatment, the role also requires strong interpersonal communication, time-management ability, and physical stamina. Therapists often spend long periods standing, demonstrating exercises, assisting with mobility tasks, and maintaining attention across multiple patient cases simultaneously. Over time, the daily responsibilities combine clinical expertise, physical activity, problem-solving, and patient coaching into a role that is both intellectually engaging and physically demanding.

Ultimately, what a physical therapist does each day depends heavily on the environment in which they practice, but the central purpose remains consistent: helping individuals regain movement, restore independence, and return to meaningful daily activities through evidence-based rehabilitation care.

2. What education is required to become a physical therapist?

Becoming a physical therapist requires completion of a **Doctor of Physical Therapy (DPT)** degree, which is the standard entry-level professional credential in the United States. Most DPT programs are structured as three-year doctoral-level professional degrees following completion of a bachelor's degree. While some students enter directly after undergraduate study, others apply after working in healthcare support roles such as rehabilitation technician, exercise specialist, athletic trainer, or personal trainer, gaining clinical exposure before formal admission.

Admission to DPT programs is competitive and typically requires completion of prerequisite coursework (gl) that includes anatomy (gl) and physiology (gl), biology, chemistry, physics, psychology, and statistics. Many programs also expect documented observation hours in physical therapy settings, allowing applicants to demonstrate exposure to the profession and confirm that they understand the realities of clinical practice. These observation experiences often become an important part of the application process because they provide early insight into whether the daily workflow of the profession aligns with the applicant's expectations.

Once admitted, DPT education combines classroom instruction, laboratory-based skill training, and extensive clinical rotations. Early coursework focuses on foundational sciences such as human anatomy, biomechanics (gl), kinesiology, neuroscience, and pathology, while later coursework emphasizes clinical examination techniques, rehabilitation intervention strategies, evidence-based practice, and specialty treatment approaches. Laboratory training allows students to practice manual techniques, movement assessments, and treatment simulations before working directly with patients in clinical environments.

Clinical education forms a substantial portion of DPT training. Students complete multiple full-time clinical rotations across different settings, such as outpatient orthopedics, inpatient rehabilitation, acute care hospitals, neurological rehabilitation programs, pediatric clinics, or specialty rehabilitation centers. These rotations allow students to experience the pace, documentation expectations, patient complexity, and interdisciplinary collaboration that define real-world practice. Exposure to multiple environments also helps students begin identifying which practice settings best match their interests and long-term career goals.

After graduation, candidates must pass the National Physical Therapy Examination (NPTE) and meet individual state licensure requirements before practicing independently. Some graduates choose to pursue postdoctoral residency or fellowship training in specialty areas such as orthopedic, neurological, sports, pediatric, or geriatric physical therapy, although these advanced programs are optional rather than required for entry-level practice.

The educational pathway is rigorous, both academically and financially, and typically represents a significant multi-year commitment. Prospective students should carefully evaluate tuition costs, projected loan repayment obligations, geographic mobility requirements for clinical placements, and long-term earning expectations before enrolling. Understanding the full scope of the educational investment helps individuals determine whether the profession aligns not only with their interests and strengths but also with their long-term financial and lifestyle planning goals.

3. How competitive is admission to physical therapy programs?

Admission to Doctor of Physical Therapy (DPT) programs is generally considered competitive, though the level of competition varies by institution, geographic region, and the number of applicants each program receives annually. Most accredited programs receive significantly more applications than available seats, meaning successful applicants typically demonstrate a combination of strong academic preparation, relevant clinical exposure, and evidence of commitment to the profession.

Grade point average remains one of the most influential components of the application process. Many programs publish minimum GPA thresholds, but meeting the minimum rarely guarantees admission. Competitive applicants often present strong performance in prerequisite science courses such as anatomy, physiology, physics, and biology, as these subjects provide early indicators of a student's ability to manage the scientific rigor of doctoral-level coursework. Admissions committees frequently evaluate not only cumulative GPA but also prerequisite GPA trends, academic improvement over time, and the overall difficulty of completed coursework.

Observation or volunteer hours in physical therapy settings are another important factor. Programs commonly require applicants to document supervised observation experiences across one or more clinical environments. These experiences help applicants confirm their understanding of the profession's daily workflow while demonstrating initiative and early professional exposure. Applicants who complete observation hours in multiple settings — such as outpatient clinics, hospitals, or rehabilitation centers — often gain a broader perspective that strengthens their application narratives and interview discussions.

Letters of recommendation also play a role in evaluating readiness for professional training. Recommendations from licensed physical therapists, academic faculty members, or healthcare supervisors provide admissions committees with insight into the applicant's professionalism, communication skills, reliability, and capacity for clinical learning. Strong letters often highlight interpersonal qualities such as teamwork, adaptability, empathy, and problem-solving ability, which are essential for clinical success but not always visible in academic transcripts.

Interviews, when included in the admissions process, allow programs to assess communication style, professional maturity, and alignment with the mission or values of the institution. Applicants may be asked to discuss why they chose the profession, how they handled challenging experiences, or what they learned during observation placements. Preparation for interviews often involves reflecting on personal motivations, ethical considerations, and long-term career goals rather than memorizing scripted responses.

While admission is competitive, it is not unattainable for applicants who prepare strategically. Strong academic performance, meaningful clinical exposure, thoughtful personal statements, and clear demonstration of commitment to the profession collectively strengthen candidacy. Prospective applicants benefit from beginning preparation early, completing prerequisite coursework carefully, gaining observation experience across different practice settings, and building professional relationships that support strong recommendations. By approaching the process deliberately rather than rushing into applications, candidates improve both admission outcomes and their own confidence in pursuing the profession with informed expectations.

4. How long does it take to become a physical therapist?

The timeline to become a licensed physical therapist typically ranges from **seven to eight years**, depending on individual educational pathways and application timing. Most individuals complete a four-year bachelor's degree followed by a three-year Doctor of Physical Therapy (DPT) program. After graduation, candidates must pass the National Physical Therapy Examination (NPTE) and meet state licensure requirements before beginning independent clinical practice, which may add several additional months depending on testing schedules and licensing timelines.

The undergraduate portion of the pathway often includes completion of prerequisite coursework required for admission to DPT programs. Students may major in exercise science, kinesiology, biology, or another health-related field, though no specific undergraduate major is universally required. What matters most is successful completion of prerequisite science courses such as anatomy, physiology, physics, chemistry, and statistics, along with observation hours completed under the supervision of licensed physical therapists. Many students use undergraduate years to gain part-time clinical experience as rehabilitation technicians or therapy aides, building familiarity with the profession while strengthening their applications.

The DPT program itself generally requires three academic years of full-time study that integrates classroom education, laboratory skill development, and clinical rotations. Clinical education becomes progressively more intensive over the course of the program, culminating in extended full-time clinical placements that allow students to function at near-entry-level clinician capacity under supervision. These rotations often occur across multiple geographic locations and practice settings, requiring flexibility and mobility during training.

After graduation, the licensing process begins. Candidates must pass the NPTE, and some states require additional jurisprudence examinations that assess knowledge of state-specific practice laws. Processing times for licensure applications vary, so new graduates often plan several months between graduation and the start of their first professional position. Once licensed, therapists may begin practicing immediately, though some choose to pursue optional residency or fellowship programs that provide additional specialty training in areas such as orthopedics, neurology, sports rehabilitation, or pediatrics. These programs typically last one year and are not required for general practice but may support advanced clinical skill development.

Although the total time commitment is significant, many individuals view the length of training as comparable to other doctoral-level healthcare professions that require advanced clinical expertise. Understanding the full timeline helps prospective students plan financially, academically, and personally for the extended educational pathway, ensuring they enter the process with realistic expectations about the years required before reaching independent clinical practice.

5. How physically demanding is the profession of physical therapy?

Physical therapy can be physically demanding, though the level of physical strain varies significantly depending on the clinical setting. Therapists frequently spend large portions of the day standing, walking between treatment areas, demonstrating exercises, assisting patients with transfers, and providing manual guidance during mobility training. In hospital, neurological, and rehabilitation environments, therapists may assist patients who require moderate physical support during walking or positioning tasks, which can contribute to cumulative musculoskeletal strain over time if body mechanics are not managed carefully.

Outpatient orthopedic clinics may involve less direct lifting but still require repeated demonstration of exercises, posture coaching, and sustained standing throughout the day. Home health and skilled nursing environments can involve additional physical demands related to working in confined spaces or assisting patients without access to mechanical lift equipment commonly found in hospitals. For these reasons, therapists often develop strong awareness of ergonomics, body mechanics, and physical conditioning strategies to maintain long-term career sustainability.

Many clinicians find the physical activity level to be a positive aspect of the profession, as the workday is rarely sedentary. However, prospective students should understand that the profession requires consistent physical engagement and should evaluate whether sustained standing, assisting mobility tasks, and demonstrating movement activities align with their long-term physical capacity and comfort.

6. What is the typical work schedule for physical therapists?

Work schedules vary widely based on practice setting. Outpatient clinics commonly operate during daytime hours but may include early-morning or evening appointments to accommodate patient work schedules. Hospital-based therapists often work standard weekday shifts, though some facilities require weekend rotations or holiday coverage depending on staffing models. Home health therapists typically manage flexible schedules organized around geographic travel routes, which may allow greater autonomy but still require full-day productivity expectations.

Inpatient rehabilitation and skilled nursing facilities usually maintain predictable weekday therapy schedules, though weekend coverage rotations are common. Specialty performance clinics or sports rehabilitation centers may operate extended hours to accommodate athletes or working clients. Telehealth and travel therapy positions may provide additional scheduling flexibility, but productivity expectations remain tied to patient visit volume and documentation completion.

Understanding scheduling differences across settings is important because work-life balance experiences vary significantly depending on the environment in which a therapist practices.

7. How much documentation is required in physical therapy practice?

Documentation is a significant component of the profession and is required for clinical communication, regulatory compliance (gl), and reimbursement justification. Therapists document initial evaluations, daily treatment notes, progress reports, discharge summaries, and communication updates related to patient care coordination. In many environments, documentation must demonstrate medical necessity, functional improvement, and measurable treatment outcomes to meet payer requirements.

The time required for documentation varies by setting and electronic health record system, but it often occupies a meaningful portion of the workday. Therapists who develop efficient charting habits — such as documenting between sessions or using structured note templates — typically experience less administrative backlog than those who postpone documentation until the end of the day. While documentation may not be the most visible aspect of the profession, it plays a critical role in care continuity and professional accountability.

8. What personality traits are helpful for success as a physical therapist?

Successful physical therapists often demonstrate a combination of communication skill, patience, problem-solving ability, and sustained interpersonal engagement. Because rehabilitation progress frequently occurs over weeks or months, therapists must maintain patient motivation even when improvements appear gradual. Clear explanation of treatment plans, consistent encouragement, and the ability to adapt communication styles to different patient populations are essential interpersonal skills.

Attention to detail is also important, as therapists must observe subtle movement changes, identify compensatory patterns, and adjust treatment strategies based on patient response. Time-management ability helps clinicians maintain schedule flow while completing documentation responsibilities, and resilience supports long-term sustainability in a profession that combines both physical and emotional demands. While individuals with many personality types can succeed in the profession, those who enjoy coaching, teaching, and working closely with people over extended recovery timelines often find strong alignment with the role.

9. Can physical therapists specialize in certain areas of practice?

Yes, physical therapists can pursue specialty certification in multiple clinical areas through professional board certification pathways. Common specialty areas include orthopedic, neurological, sports, pediatric, geriatric, cardiovascular and pulmonary, oncologic, and women's health physical therapy. Specialization typically involves accumulating clinical experience in the chosen area, completing advanced continuing education, and passing a specialty certification examination administered by professional credentialing bodies.

Specialization can support career advancement, expand clinical expertise, and sometimes open opportunities for leadership, teaching, or advanced clinical roles. While specialty certification is not required for practice, many clinicians pursue it after gaining several years of experience to deepen expertise in patient populations that align most closely with their professional interests.

10. What is the job outlook for physical therapists?

The job outlook for physical therapists is generally strong and is driven by several long-term healthcare trends, including population aging, increased survival following traumatic injuries and complex medical conditions, and growing recognition of rehabilitation's role in improving long-term functional outcomes. As more individuals live longer and remain active later in life, demand for rehabilitation services related to orthopedic conditions, balance impairments, neurological disorders, and post-surgical recovery continues to expand.

In addition to aging demographics, healthcare systems increasingly emphasize mobility preservation, fall prevention, and non-pharmacological pain management strategies, all of which involve rehabilitation professionals. Expanding outpatient rehabilitation networks, home health services, and community-based care models also contribute to ongoing workforce demand. However, employment conditions can vary regionally, with some geographic areas experiencing higher demand than others, particularly rural or underserved communities where clinician shortages are more common.

Overall, while workforce demand does fluctuate with reimbursement policies and healthcare system restructuring, physical therapy remains a profession with relatively stable long-term employment opportunities compared to many other healthcare roles.

11. How much do physical therapists earn?

Compensation for physical therapists varies based on geographic region, clinical setting, years of experience, and specialization. Therapists working in outpatient clinics, hospitals, rehabilitation centers, home health agencies, or specialty performance environments may experience different salary structures, with some settings offering productivity-based incentives or performance bonuses tied to patient volume or service delivery metrics.

Early-career therapists typically begin at entry-level salary ranges that increase gradually with experience, additional certifications, or leadership responsibilities such as clinical supervision, program development, or department management. Travel therapy positions may offer higher short-term compensation packages due to staffing shortages or temporary placement incentives, though these roles may involve geographic mobility and variable contract durations.

When evaluating compensation, it is important to consider the full financial picture, including benefits, retirement contributions, continuing education support, schedule flexibility, and long-term earning trajectory rather than focusing only on starting salary figures. Because education costs for doctoral-level programs can be significant, prospective students should evaluate projected loan repayment obligations alongside expected compensation ranges to ensure long-term financial sustainability.

12. Is physical therapy a good long-term career?

Whether physical therapy is a strong long-term career depends largely on alignment between the profession's daily demands and an individual's preferred work style, physical capacity, and career expectations. Many clinicians find long-term satisfaction in helping patients regain independence, observing measurable recovery progress, and working in environments that emphasize functional improvement rather than short-term procedural interventions.

At the same time, long-term career sustainability often depends on choosing the right practice setting. Some clinicians eventually transition into specialty practice, administrative leadership, teaching roles, research positions, or hybrid clinical-management roles as their careers progress. Others move into consulting, ergonomics, workplace injury prevention, or rehabilitation program design. These career pathways allow professionals to remain within the rehabilitation field while adjusting workload intensity or clinical focus over time.

Understanding that the profession offers multiple career evolution pathways helps individuals evaluate physical therapy not only as an entry-level clinical role but also as a platform for long-term professional development across diverse healthcare environments.

13. What types of patients do physical therapists treat?

Physical therapists work with a wide range of patient populations across the lifespan, from infants with developmental delays to older adults recovering from surgery, injury, or chronic health conditions. Common patient categories include individuals recovering from orthopedic injuries, joint replacement surgeries, neurological conditions such as stroke or spinal cord injury, cardiopulmonary illness affecting endurance and mobility, sports-related injuries, and chronic pain disorders that impact daily function.

Treatment approaches vary based on patient needs, ranging from exercise-based rehabilitation and balance training to mobility retraining, endurance conditioning, functional task practice, and education focused on injury prevention. Therapists also work closely with interdisciplinary teams that may include physicians, occupational therapists, speech-language pathologists, nurses, athletic trainers, and case managers to coordinate comprehensive care plans.

The diversity of patient populations is one of the defining features of the profession, offering clinicians opportunities to explore different specialty areas and practice environments over the course of their careers.

14. What is the difference between a physical therapist and a physical therapist assistant?

Physical therapists (PTs) and physical therapist assistants (PTAs) work closely together but have different educational pathways, scopes of responsibility, and clinical decision-making authority. Physical therapists complete doctoral-level education and are responsible for performing initial patient evaluations, establishing treatment plans, modifying care strategies, and completing discharge assessments. They also supervise delegated components of care delivered by PTAs and therapy aides.

Physical therapist assistants typically complete associate-degree-level education programs and provide treatment interventions under the supervision of a licensed physical therapist. PTAs may guide patients through prescribed exercises, assist with mobility training, and document treatment sessions, but they do not independently perform initial evaluations or develop treatment plans. The collaborative PT–PTA relationship allows rehabilitation teams to deliver efficient patient care while maintaining professional oversight and coordinated treatment progression.

15. Do physical therapists spend most of their time exercising with patients?

While exercise instruction is a central part of the profession, the role involves far more than simply guiding workouts. Physical therapists evaluate movement patterns, identify biomechanical or neurological impairments, design individualized treatment plans, monitor patient response, and adjust interventions based on clinical progress. Sessions may include manual therapy techniques, balance training, mobility retraining, patient education, and functional activity practice in addition to therapeutic exercise. Documentation, interdisciplinary communication, and care planning also occupy a meaningful portion of the workday. The balance between hands-on treatment and administrative responsibilities varies by practice setting, but clinical reasoning and patient coaching remain constant components of daily work.

16. How much student loan debt do physical therapy graduates typically carry?

Student loan debt varies widely depending on tuition costs, residency status, scholarships, and whether students attend public or private institutions. Because the Doctor of Physical Therapy degree is a doctoral-level program requiring multiple years of full-time study, total educational borrowing can be significant for some graduates. Prospective students are encouraged to calculate projected total tuition, living expenses, and anticipated loan repayment amounts before enrolling, comparing those figures with expected entry-level salaries and long-term earning potential. Many clinicians manage debt successfully through income-driven repayment plans, employer-sponsored loan assistance programs, or geographic job selection strategies that allow accelerated repayment early in their careers.

17. Can physical therapists open their own clinics?

Yes, many physical therapists eventually pursue private practice ownership after gaining clinical experience and developing business management knowledge. Opening a clinic involves responsibilities beyond patient care, including regulatory compliance, payer contracting, staffing, marketing, financial management, and operational planning. Some therapists begin by working as employees, later transitioning into partnership models or independent ownership once they understand reimbursement systems and patient acquisition strategies. While entrepreneurship offers autonomy and income potential, it also introduces administrative responsibilities that differ significantly from purely clinical roles, making business preparation an important step for those considering private practice pathways.

18. Is burnout common in physical therapy?

Burnout risk varies by workplace environment, productivity expectations, documentation workload, and alignment between the clinician's work style and practice setting. Therapists working in high-volume environments with limited schedule flexibility may experience higher stress if administrative demands and patient throughput expectations consistently exceed manageable workflow capacity. However, clinicians who select practice settings aligned with their preferences—such as home health, specialty rehabilitation, academic roles, or performance training environments—often report strong long-term career satisfaction. Career sustainability frequently depends less on the profession itself and more on the conditions under which the work is performed, highlighting the importance of thoughtful setting selection early in one's career.

19. Do physical therapists work as part of healthcare teams?

Yes, physical therapists routinely function as members of interdisciplinary healthcare teams that may include physicians, nurses, occupational therapists, speech-language pathologists, case managers, athletic trainers, psychologists, and social workers. Collaboration is particularly important in hospital, rehabilitation, neurological, and pediatric settings where coordinated care plans determine discharge readiness and long-term recovery outcomes. Effective communication with team members ensures treatment goals remain aligned, patient safety considerations are addressed, and functional progress is integrated into the broader medical plan of care. Strong teamwork skills are therefore essential professional competencies in most rehabilitation environments.

20. What settings can physical therapists work in?

Physical therapists work across a wide range of healthcare and performance environments, allowing significant career flexibility over time. Common practice settings include outpatient orthopedic clinics, hospitals, inpatient rehabilitation facilities, home health agencies, skilled nursing facilities, pediatric centers, sports performance clinics, academic medical centers, and community-based wellness or prevention programs. Some therapists also work in specialized roles within occupational health programs, military rehabilitation systems, professional sports organizations, research institutions, or telehealth-based care models. Because many clinicians change settings at different stages of their careers, the profession offers multiple pathways for adjusting workload intensity, patient population, or lifestyle preferences without leaving the field entirely.

21. Is physical therapy emotionally demanding?

Physical therapy can be emotionally demanding, particularly when working with patients recovering from traumatic injuries, chronic illnesses, or life-changing medical events. Therapists often support individuals who are navigating pain, loss of independence, or uncertainty about long-term recovery, requiring strong communication skills and emotional resilience. At the same time, many clinicians find deep professional meaning in witnessing patient progress and helping individuals regain functional independence. Emotional demands tend to vary by setting, with acute care and neurological rehabilitation environments often involving higher exposure to complex medical situations, while outpatient and performance-focused environments may involve different types of motivational challenges. Developing professional boundaries and effective coping strategies is an important part of long-term career sustainability.

22. How important is patient motivation in physical therapy outcomes?

Patient motivation plays a critical role in rehabilitation outcomes because progress depends heavily on consistent participation in treatment sessions and adherence to prescribed home exercise programs. Physical therapists frequently act as coaches, helping patients understand the purpose of exercises, track progress milestones, and maintain engagement throughout recovery timelines that may extend over weeks or months. Therapists also adapt treatment strategies when motivation declines, adjusting goals to remain realistic and achievable. While clinical skill and treatment design are essential, patient engagement often determines how effectively rehabilitation plans translate into functional improvement outside the clinic setting.

23. Are there opportunities for advancement in physical therapy careers?

Yes, physical therapy offers multiple advancement pathways beyond entry-level clinical practice. Clinicians may pursue specialty certifications (gl), clinical leadership roles, department management positions, teaching appointments within academic programs, research careers, or consulting roles in ergonomics, injury prevention, and rehabilitation program design. Some therapists transition into healthcare administration, clinical education coordination, or private practice ownership. Advancement opportunities often depend on gaining experience, developing specialized expertise, and building professional networks that support leadership or academic transitions over time.

24. How portable is a physical therapy license between states?

Physical therapy licensure is issued at the state level, meaning therapists must hold a valid license in each state where they practice. However, many jurisdictions participate in licensure portability agreements that allow clinicians to obtain practice privileges in multiple participating states through streamlined application processes. Requirements vary, and therapists planning to relocate or work in travel positions often research state-specific regulations in advance to ensure smooth licensure transitions. Maintaining continuing education requirements (gl) and keeping licensure credentials current is essential for preserving practice eligibility across jurisdictions.

25. Do physical therapists need continuing education to maintain their licenses?

Yes. Most states require licensed physical therapists to complete continuing education credits on a recurring basis to maintain licensure. These requirements ensure clinicians remain current with evolving treatment techniques, safety standards, and evidence-based practice updates. Continuing education may include formal coursework, clinical workshops, specialty certification training, or approved professional conferences. Therapists often select courses aligned with their practice setting or specialty interests, allowing continuing education to function not only as a regulatory requirement but also as a long-term professional development strategy.

26. Can physical therapists change specialties during their careers?

Yes. One of the advantages of the profession is the ability to transition between practice settings over time. A therapist may begin in outpatient orthopedics, later move into neurological rehabilitation, home health care, sports performance, pediatrics, or academic roles depending on evolving interests and lifestyle needs. Some transitions require additional continuing education or mentorship to develop confidence in new clinical areas, but formal retraining programs are not always necessary. This flexibility allows clinicians to adjust workload intensity, patient populations, or career focus without leaving the rehabilitation field entirely.

27. How important are communication skills in physical therapy?

Communication skills are central to effective physical therapy practice. Therapists must explain treatment plans clearly, teach exercise techniques, provide feedback on movement quality, and motivate patients who may feel discouraged during recovery. They also communicate regularly with physicians, nurses, case managers, and other healthcare professionals to coordinate patient care. Strong listening skills are equally important, as understanding patient concerns, goals, and barriers to participation helps therapists tailor treatment plans that are realistic and sustainable. Clear communication improves adherence, safety, and long-term rehabilitation outcomes.

28. What challenges do new graduate physical therapists commonly face?

New graduates often face a transition period in which they adapt from structured academic training to full clinical responsibility. Common challenges include managing larger patient caseloads, completing documentation efficiently, developing confidence in independent clinical decision-making, and learning workplace-specific workflow systems. Time-management skills typically improve within the first year as therapists become more familiar with treatment planning, charting expectations, and interdisciplinary communication processes. Mentorship from experienced clinicians during early career stages can significantly ease this transition and accelerate professional confidence.

29. Is it possible to work part-time as a physical therapist?

Yes. Many practice settings offer part-time or flexible scheduling arrangements, particularly outpatient clinics, home health agencies, telehealth services, and some rehabilitation facilities. Part-time roles may appeal to clinicians balancing family responsibilities, pursuing academic study, operating private businesses, or gradually transitioning toward retirement. Compensation structures and benefit eligibility may differ for part-time positions, so therapists typically evaluate schedule flexibility alongside financial considerations when choosing reduced-hour roles. Flexible scheduling options contribute to the profession's adaptability across different life stages.

30. Do physical therapists work weekends or holidays?

Weekend or holiday work depends largely on the practice setting. Hospital-based therapists, inpatient rehabilitation facilities, and skilled nursing environments often maintain weekend coverage rotations to ensure patient mobility and discharge planning continue without interruption. Outpatient clinics typically operate Monday through Friday, although some offer weekend appointments to accommodate patient schedules. Home health therapists may have greater scheduling flexibility but still manage productivity expectations that may occasionally include weekend visits. Understanding scheduling patterns across settings helps clinicians select work environments aligned with their preferred work-life balance.

31. How important is teamwork in physical therapy practice?

Teamwork is a fundamental component of physical therapy practice, particularly in hospital, rehabilitation, pediatric, and neurological care environments where coordinated interdisciplinary treatment plans determine patient outcomes. Therapists regularly collaborate with physicians, nurses, occupational therapists, speech-language pathologists, case managers, and social workers to ensure mobility goals align with broader medical treatment plans. Effective teamwork improves care continuity, reduces safety risks, and helps patients transition smoothly between levels of care.

32. Can physical therapists work internationally?

Physical therapists may work internationally, but licensure requirements vary by country. Clinicians seeking international employment typically must meet credential recognition standards established by the destination country, which may involve credential evaluation, additional examinations, language proficiency requirements, or supervised practice periods. Some international positions are available through global healthcare organizations, military systems, or humanitarian service programs. Therapists interested in international practice often research regulatory requirements early to plan credential portability effectively.

33. Do physical therapists use technology in their daily work?

Yes. Modern physical therapy practice incorporates electronic health record systems, outcome-tracking software, telehealth platforms, wearable movement-monitoring technology, and rehabilitation equipment that provides objective performance data. Technology supports documentation efficiency, treatment planning, remote patient monitoring, and evidence-based clinical decision-making. As digital healthcare systems continue evolving, familiarity with clinical technology platforms becomes an increasingly important professional competency.

34. What role does evidence-based practice play in physical therapy?

Evidence-based practice is a central principle of the profession and involves integrating clinical expertise, patient preferences, and the best available research evidence when designing treatment plans. Therapists regularly review clinical guidelines, research literature, and outcome data to determine which interventions are most appropriate for specific patient populations. Continuing education courses, professional conferences, and specialty certification programs often emphasize evidence-based treatment updates, ensuring clinicians remain current with evolving rehabilitation science. Applying evidence-based principles helps improve patient outcomes, supports professional credibility, and aligns clinical practice with modern healthcare quality standards.

35. Is physical therapy a stressful career?

Stress levels in physical therapy vary by practice setting, productivity expectations, documentation workload, and workplace culture. Clinicians working in high-volume outpatient clinics or fast-paced hospital environments may experience time pressure when balancing patient care responsibilities with administrative requirements. However, therapists who work in settings aligned with their preferred pace—such as home health, specialty rehabilitation programs, or academic roles—often report more manageable stress levels. Long-term career satisfaction is frequently influenced less by the profession itself and more by whether the chosen workplace environment fits the clinician's workflow preferences, physical stamina, and long-term lifestyle priorities.

36. Do physical therapists treat only injuries?

No. While injury rehabilitation is a major component of the profession, physical therapists also treat chronic medical conditions, neurological disorders, developmental delays, balance impairments, cardiopulmonary limitations, and mobility challenges related to aging or long-term illness. Many therapists also focus on injury prevention, performance optimization, ergonomic education, and wellness programs designed to reduce future functional decline. The profession therefore extends beyond injury recovery into long-term functional health management across the lifespan.

37. How important is physical fitness for physical therapists?

Maintaining personal physical fitness can be helpful because the profession often involves sustained standing, demonstration of exercises, assisting patients with movement, and maintaining energy throughout a full clinical day. While therapists are not required to maintain athletic-level fitness, basic strength, mobility, and endurance support long-term musculoskeletal health and reduce occupational strain. Many clinicians adopt regular stretching, strengthening, and conditioning routines to sustain physical resilience throughout their careers.

38. Can physical therapists move into non-clinical careers?

Yes. Some physical therapists transition into non-clinical roles such as healthcare administration, rehabilitation program management, medical device consulting, ergonomics consulting, insurance utilization review, healthcare policy work, clinical education, or academic teaching positions. These transitions often occur after clinicians gain several years of clinical experience and develop expertise that translates into leadership, consulting, or system-level healthcare roles. The profession's foundation in movement science and patient care provides transferable skills applicable to a variety of healthcare-related career pathways.

39. Do physical therapists work with athletes?

Yes. Many physical therapists specialize in sports rehabilitation and performance training, working with athletes ranging from youth competitors to professional sports teams. Treatment in these environments focuses on injury recovery, movement analysis, performance optimization, and injury-prevention training. Collaboration with athletic trainers, strength and conditioning coaches, and team physicians is common. While sports rehabilitation is a popular career interest among students, available positions are often competitive, making clinical experience, networking, and specialty certification important steps for clinicians pursuing this pathway.

40. Do physical therapists need strong science backgrounds?

Yes. Physical therapy education relies heavily on foundational sciences such as anatomy, physiology, biomechanics, neuroscience, and pathology. Understanding how muscles, joints, nerves, and body systems function allows therapists to evaluate movement impairments accurately and design effective rehabilitation strategies. While students do not need to begin their education as science experts, comfort with learning scientific material and applying it to clinical problem-solving is essential for success in DPT programs and professional practice.

41. Can physical therapists work with children?

Yes. Pediatric physical therapists specialize in treating infants, children, and adolescents with developmental delays, congenital conditions, neurological disorders, orthopedic injuries, or mobility challenges related to chronic health conditions. Treatment often incorporates play-based activities designed to improve strength, coordination, balance, and functional mobility while maintaining engagement appropriate for the child's developmental stage. Pediatric therapists frequently collaborate with families, teachers, occupational therapists, and speech-language pathologists to coordinate comprehensive developmental care.

42. How important is manual therapy in physical therapy?

Manual therapy, which includes hands-on techniques such as joint mobilization, soft tissue work, and guided movement assistance, is one of many tools used in rehabilitation. While some practice settings emphasize manual therapy more heavily than others, most treatment programs combine hands-on techniques with exercise-based interventions, functional training, and patient education. The importance of manual therapy varies depending on patient condition, therapist training, and clinical setting, but it remains a commonly used component of comprehensive rehabilitation care.

43. Do physical therapists have opportunities to teach?

Yes. Many physical therapists participate in teaching roles throughout their careers, whether by supervising students during clinical rotations, providing continuing education courses, teaching within academic DPT programs, or leading community injury-prevention workshops. Clinicians who pursue academic careers often complete additional graduate-level education or develop research experience to qualify for faculty positions. Teaching opportunities allow therapists to contribute to professional development while expanding their own clinical expertise.

44. Is relocation common in physical therapy careers?

Relocation is not required, but some clinicians choose to relocate early in their careers to access preferred practice settings, higher-demand geographic regions, or specialized training opportunities. Travel therapy assignments also provide short-term relocation experiences for clinicians interested in working in multiple regions over time. Because licensure requirements vary by state, therapists planning relocation typically research licensing processes in advance to ensure a smooth transition between jurisdictions.

45. Do physical therapists work with older adults?

Yes. A significant portion of physical therapy practice involves working with older adults who are managing mobility limitations related to aging, chronic health conditions, joint replacement surgeries, balance impairments, or fall risk. Treatment often focuses on improving walking safety, strengthening muscles that support functional independence, enhancing balance, and helping individuals maintain the ability to perform daily activities. Therapists working in geriatric (gl) settings frequently collaborate with caregivers and interdisciplinary teams to support long-term independence and quality of life.

46. Can physical therapists treat neurological conditions?

Yes. Many physical therapists specialize in neurological rehabilitation, treating individuals recovering from stroke, traumatic brain injury (gl), spinal cord injury, Parkinson's disease, multiple sclerosis, and other neurological conditions affecting movement and coordination. Treatment emphasizes motor retraining, balance work, gait restoration, endurance building, and adaptive movement strategies that help patients regain functional independence. Neurological rehabilitation often requires patience and long-term treatment planning because recovery may occur gradually over extended periods.

47. Is private practice ownership common in physical therapy?

Private practice ownership is a common long-term career pathway for therapists who develop clinical expertise and business management skills. Owners are responsible not only for patient care but also for operational responsibilities such as staffing, financial management, regulatory compliance, marketing, and payer contracting. Some clinicians open independent clinics, while others join partnership models or expand into multi-location rehabilitation organizations. Entrepreneurship can provide increased autonomy and income potential, though it also introduces additional administrative responsibilities beyond clinical care.

48. How important is time management in physical therapy?

Time management is a critical professional skill because therapists must balance patient treatment sessions, documentation requirements, interdisciplinary communication, and care planning responsibilities within structured daily schedules. Efficient workflow habits—such as documenting between sessions, preparing treatment plans in advance, and organizing patient materials—help clinicians maintain productivity while reducing after-hours administrative workload. Strong time-management ability contributes significantly to long-term career sustainability and workplace satisfaction.

49. Do physical therapists have opportunities for leadership roles?

Yes. Experienced physical therapists may move into leadership positions such as clinical supervisors, department managers, rehabilitation directors, program coordinators, academic faculty members, or professional association leaders. Leadership roles often involve mentoring staff, overseeing clinical operations, developing treatment programs, and participating in organizational decision-making. Advancement into leadership positions typically follows several years of clinical experience combined with demonstrated organizational, communication, and management skills.

50. Are physical therapists involved in discharge planning?

Yes. In hospital and rehabilitation settings, physical therapists play a key role in discharge planning by evaluating a patient's mobility level, safety with daily activities, and need for ongoing rehabilitation services. Therapists provide recommendations regarding whether patients can safely return home, require home health therapy, benefit from outpatient rehabilitation, or need transfer to inpatient rehabilitation facilities. These recommendations help case managers, physicians, and families make informed decisions that support safe transitions of care and reduce the risk of readmission.

51. Can physical therapists work in research?

Yes. Some physical therapists pursue careers in clinical or academic research, studying rehabilitation outcomes, movement science, injury prevention strategies, and evidence-based treatment approaches. Research roles may exist within universities, healthcare systems, government agencies, or private research organizations. Clinicians interested in research often pursue advanced academic degrees or collaborate with research teams while maintaining part-time clinical practice. Research contributions help advance rehabilitation science and improve long-term patient care standards.

52. What role does patient education play in physical therapy?

Patient education is a central component of rehabilitation care. Therapists teach patients how to perform exercises correctly, manage activity levels safely, understand recovery timelines, and adopt movement habits that reduce reinjury risk. Because patients spend most of their time outside therapy sessions, their ability to apply these strategies independently strongly influences long-term recovery outcomes. Clear communication, demonstration, and reinforcement of home exercise programs are therefore essential elements of daily practice.

53. Do physical therapists use outcome measures to track progress?

Yes. Physical therapists routinely use standardized outcome measures to evaluate patient progress, assess functional improvement, and guide treatment decision-making. These tools may include mobility tests, balance assessments, strength measurements, endurance evaluations, and patient-reported functional surveys. Tracking measurable outcomes allows clinicians to determine whether treatment strategies are effective and provides objective data required for documentation, reimbursement justification, and interdisciplinary care coordination.

54. Can physical therapists work in community wellness or prevention programs?

Yes. Some physical therapists work in community-based wellness initiatives focused on fall prevention, injury prevention, mobility screening, workplace ergonomics, and health promotion programs designed to maintain functional independence across populations. These roles may involve partnerships with community organizations, employers, schools, or public health agencies. Prevention-focused practice allows therapists to apply rehabilitation expertise proactively rather than only after injury or illness occurs.

55. Do physical therapists need strong problem-solving skills?

Yes. Physical therapy requires continuous clinical problem-solving because each patient presents with unique movement limitations, medical histories, and recovery responses. Therapists evaluate how impairments affect functional activities, determine which interventions are most appropriate, and adjust treatment plans based on patient progress or changing medical status. Strong analytical thinking allows clinicians to identify underlying causes of movement dysfunction rather than treating symptoms alone, improving long-term rehabilitation outcomes.

56. Can physical therapists work with patients who have chronic illnesses?

Yes. Many therapists work with patients managing chronic conditions such as arthritis, cardiovascular disease, pulmonary disorders, neurological illnesses, and long-term pain syndromes. Treatment often focuses on improving endurance, mobility, strength, and activity tolerance while teaching pacing strategies that help patients manage symptoms safely. Rehabilitation for chronic illness frequently emphasizes long-term functional maintenance rather than short-term recovery alone.

57. How important is adaptability in physical therapy practice?

Adaptability is essential because therapists regularly work with patients whose conditions, tolerance levels, and recovery trajectories change over time. Treatment plans often require modification based on new symptoms, surgical updates, or unexpected progress variations. Therapists also adapt to different workplace environments, electronic record systems, interdisciplinary teams, and scheduling demands. Flexibility in clinical reasoning (gl) and workflow management supports effective care delivery across diverse settings.

58. Do physical therapists interact with insurance companies?

Yes. While therapists may not always communicate directly with insurance representatives, clinical documentation must meet payer requirements that demonstrate medical necessity, treatment effectiveness, and functional improvement. In some settings, therapists participate in authorization requests, peer-to-peer clinical reviews, or appeals processes to justify ongoing treatment services. Understanding reimbursement requirements is therefore an important administrative aspect of professional practice.

59. Can physical therapists participate in professional organizations?

Yes. Many therapists join professional organizations that provide continuing education opportunities, clinical resources, networking events, advocacy initiatives, and specialty certification pathways. Participation in professional associations supports ongoing professional development, helps clinicians remain informed about regulatory changes affecting the profession, and offers leadership opportunities at regional or national levels.

60. Do physical therapists need strong observational skills?

Yes. Physical therapists rely heavily on observational skills to identify subtle movement abnormalities, compensatory patterns, balance deficits, and posture changes that may not be immediately obvious to patients. Careful observation allows clinicians to refine diagnoses, adjust treatment techniques, and monitor functional progress accurately over time. Strong observational ability supports safer treatment progression and more precise rehabilitation planning.

61. Can physical therapists work in rehabilitation technology development?

Yes. Some physical therapists collaborate with technology companies, research institutions, or healthcare innovation teams to help design rehabilitation equipment, wearable movement-monitoring devices, virtual rehabilitation platforms, and digital therapy programs. Clinical expertise allows therapists to contribute valuable insight into how technology can be used safely and effectively in real-world patient care environments.

62. How important is cultural competence in physical therapy practice?

Cultural competence is increasingly important because therapists work with patients from diverse backgrounds with varying health beliefs, communication styles, and access to care resources. Understanding cultural differences helps clinicians tailor education strategies, build trust, and design treatment plans that align with patient lifestyles and expectations. Effective culturally responsive care improves patient engagement and rehabilitation outcomes.

63. Do physical therapists provide preventive care services?

Yes. In addition to treating existing injuries and conditions, many therapists provide preventive services such as ergonomic assessments, fall-risk screenings, workplace injury-prevention programs, posture education, and movement analysis designed to reduce future injury risk. Preventive care roles are expanding as healthcare systems increasingly emphasize long-term functional health maintenance.

64. Can physical therapists mentor students or new graduates?

Yes. Experienced physical therapists frequently mentor students during clinical rotations and provide onboarding support for new graduate clinicians entering the workforce. Mentorship may include guidance on clinical reasoning, documentation efficiency, patient communication strategies, and career development planning. Strong mentorship relationships play an important role in developing confident early-career clinicians and maintaining professional standards across the field.

65. Do physical therapists need strong interpersonal skills?

Yes. Interpersonal skills are central to effective rehabilitation because therapists work closely with patients over repeated treatment sessions, often building therapeutic relationships that support motivation and long-term adherence to treatment plans. Clear communication, empathy, patience, and the ability to encourage individuals during challenging recovery periods all contribute to successful outcomes. Therapists also interact frequently with interdisciplinary team members, making professional communication an essential competency across clinical environments.

66. Can physical therapists work in home health settings?

Yes. Home health physical therapists provide rehabilitation services directly in patients' homes, often working with individuals recovering from surgery, managing chronic conditions, or experiencing mobility limitations that make clinic visits difficult. Treatment in the home environment allows therapists to evaluate real-life mobility challenges such as stair navigation, bathroom safety, and household movement tasks. Home health practice typically involves travel between patient locations and independent schedule management, requiring strong organizational skills.

67. How important is documentation accuracy in physical therapy?

Accurate documentation is essential because treatment notes serve as legal records of care, communication tools for interdisciplinary teams, and evidence supporting reimbursement for therapy services. Documentation must clearly describe patient condition, treatment interventions, functional progress, and clinical justification for ongoing therapy. Precise charting supports continuity of care and protects both the clinician and healthcare organization in regulatory or legal review situations.

68. Can physical therapists work in administrative roles?

Yes. Some clinicians transition into administrative positions such as rehabilitation department managers, clinical operations directors, program coordinators, or healthcare system leadership roles. Administrative responsibilities may include staffing oversight, budgeting, quality improvement initiatives, regulatory compliance (gl) monitoring, and strategic program development. Many therapists move into these roles after gaining several years of clinical experience and demonstrating leadership capability.

69. Do physical therapists participate in interdisciplinary care planning?

Yes. Physical therapists routinely contribute to interdisciplinary care planning meetings where healthcare professionals collaborate to determine treatment priorities, discharge readiness, and long-term care needs. Their mobility and functional assessment findings help guide decisions about assistive devices, rehabilitation placement, home safety requirements, and caregiver training needs. Participation in team-based planning ensures rehabilitation goals remain integrated within the overall medical treatment plan.

70. Do physical therapists work with patients recovering from surgery?

Yes. Post-surgical rehabilitation is a major component of physical therapy practice. Therapists help patients regain mobility, rebuild strength, restore joint range of motion, and return safely to daily activities following procedures such as joint replacements, ligament repairs, spinal surgeries, or fracture repairs. Treatment plans are typically structured around surgical protocols while being individualized to each patient's recovery pace and functional goals.

71. Can physical therapists help prevent falls?

Yes. Fall-prevention programs are a key area of practice, particularly for older adults or individuals with balance impairments, neurological conditions, or mobility limitations. Therapists evaluate walking stability, strength, environmental hazards, and assistive device needs, then design interventions that improve balance, reaction time, and safe mobility. Education on home safety modifications is often included to reduce fall risk outside the clinical environment.

72. How important is patient trust in physical therapy outcomes?

Patient trust plays a critical role in rehabilitation success because treatment often requires individuals to attempt movements that feel uncomfortable or challenging during recovery. When patients trust their therapist's guidance, they are more likely to participate fully in treatment sessions, adhere to home exercise programs, and communicate openly about symptoms or concerns. Strong therapeutic relationships support consistent engagement and long-term recovery progress.

73. Can physical therapists work in academic teaching roles?

Yes. Many physical therapists serve as faculty members in Doctor of Physical Therapy programs or participate as adjunct instructors teaching clinical skills, rehabilitation science, or professional practice courses. Academic roles may involve classroom instruction, laboratory teaching, student mentoring, research participation, and curriculum development. Faculty positions often require advanced academic credentials and clinical experience.

74. Do physical therapists contribute to quality improvement initiatives?

Yes. Therapists frequently participate in healthcare quality improvement projects aimed at improving patient outcomes, reducing hospital readmissions, enhancing mobility protocols, and increasing rehabilitation efficiency. These initiatives may involve outcome data analysis, workflow redesign, interdisciplinary collaboration, and implementation of evidence-based clinical pathways that improve care delivery across healthcare systems.

5. Do physical therapists need strong teaching abilities?

Yes. Teaching is a daily component of physical therapy practice because clinicians must instruct patients on exercise techniques, movement strategies, safety precautions, and self-management skills that support recovery outside formal treatment sessions. Effective teaching involves clear demonstration, simplified explanations, and repetition that helps patients perform exercises independently with correct technique. Strong educational skills improve adherence to treatment programs and contribute significantly to long-term functional outcomes.

76. Can physical therapists work in consulting roles?

Yes. Some experienced clinicians work as consultants in areas such as ergonomics, workplace injury prevention, rehabilitation program design, healthcare operations improvement, and medical device development. Consulting roles may involve collaboration with employers, healthcare organizations, or technology companies seeking expertise in movement science and injury prevention strategies. These opportunities often emerge after clinicians develop specialized knowledge and professional networks within the field.

77. How important is professional networking in physical therapy careers?

Professional networking can influence career advancement, specialty training opportunities, mentorship relationships, and leadership development. Connections formed through clinical workplaces, professional associations, continuing education courses, and academic programs often lead to job opportunities or collaborative projects. Networking also helps clinicians stay informed about emerging clinical practices and evolving healthcare trends.

78. Do physical therapists need leadership skills?

Leadership skills become increasingly important as therapists advance in their careers, particularly when supervising support staff, mentoring students, coordinating interdisciplinary care teams, or managing clinical departments. Leadership abilities include communication, conflict resolution, organizational planning, and the ability to guide teams toward shared patient-care goals. Even early-career therapists benefit from developing leadership competencies that support collaborative practice environments.

79. Can physical therapists work in humanitarian or disaster response programs?

Yes. Some physical therapists participate in humanitarian healthcare missions, global rehabilitation initiatives, or disaster response programs where mobility restoration and injury recovery services are needed following natural disasters or humanitarian crises. These roles may involve collaboration with international aid organizations and require adaptability to resource-limited environments while delivering essential rehabilitation care.

80. Do physical therapists help patients return to work?

Yes. Many physical therapists assist patients in safely returning to work following injury, surgery, or illness by restoring strength, endurance, and functional mobility needed for job-specific tasks. In some settings, therapists perform functional capacity evaluations that measure lifting ability, movement tolerance, and physical readiness for occupational duties. They may also provide ergonomic recommendations or graded return-to-work conditioning programs that help individuals transition back to employment safely.

81. Can physical therapists work with individuals experiencing chronic pain?

Yes. Chronic pain management is a significant area of practice in which therapists help patients improve movement tolerance, rebuild strength gradually, and learn pacing strategies that reduce symptom flare-ups. Treatment often combines education, exercise progression, and behavioral movement strategies designed to restore confidence in daily activity participation. Chronic pain rehabilitation frequently emphasizes long-term functional improvement rather than immediate symptom elimination.

82. How important is continuing professional growth in physical therapy?

Continuing professional growth is essential because rehabilitation science evolves continuously, introducing new treatment approaches, technology, and clinical research findings. Therapists maintain professional competence through continuing education courses, specialty certifications, conferences, and evidence-based literature review. Lifelong learning supports improved patient outcomes and enhances career advancement opportunities.

83. Do physical therapists use assistive devices during treatment?

Yes. Therapists frequently evaluate and train patients in the use of assistive devices such as walkers, canes, crutches, braces, and mobility supports designed to improve safety and independence. Proper device selection, fitting, and patient instruction are critical components of mobility training, particularly for individuals recovering from surgery, injury, or neurological conditions affecting balance.

84. Can physical therapists work in telehealth environments?

Yes. Telehealth rehabilitation services allow therapists to evaluate movement patterns, guide exercise programs, provide education, and monitor patient progress remotely using secure digital platforms. Telehealth practice expands access to care for patients living in remote areas or those with transportation limitations, while still requiring careful communication, observation, and clinical judgment to ensure treatment safety and effectiveness.

85. Do physical therapists help patients improve balance and coordination?

Yes. Improving balance and coordination is a central component of many rehabilitation programs, particularly for older adults, individuals recovering from neurological conditions, and patients returning to activity following injury or surgery. Therapists design progressive balance exercises, walking drills, and functional movement activities that improve stability and reduce fall risk. These interventions are often combined with strength training and environmental safety education to support long-term mobility independence.

86. Can physical therapists treat patients with cardiovascular or pulmonary conditions?

Yes. Some physical therapists specialize in cardiovascular and pulmonary rehabilitation, working with patients recovering from heart surgery, cardiac events, chronic lung disease, or reduced endurance related to medical illness. Treatment focuses on monitored exercise progression, breathing techniques, endurance training, and education that supports safe activity participation while improving overall functional capacity.

87. How important is ethical decision-making in physical therapy practice?

Ethical decision-making is essential because therapists must consistently prioritize patient safety, informed consent, professional boundaries, and responsible clinical judgment when determining treatment strategies. Ethical considerations also guide documentation practices, patient confidentiality, and collaboration with healthcare teams. Adhering to professional ethical standards protects patients, clinicians, and healthcare organizations while maintaining trust in the profession.

88. Do physical therapists evaluate posture and movement patterns?

Yes. Evaluation of posture, movement mechanics, and functional mobility is a fundamental component of physical therapy assessment. Therapists analyze how patients move during daily activities, identify compensatory patterns that contribute to pain or dysfunction, and design treatment strategies that restore efficient movement patterns. Movement analysis supports targeted rehabilitation interventions that address underlying causes rather than symptoms alone.

89. Can physical therapists work with individuals who have disabilities?

Yes. Physical therapists frequently work with individuals who have temporary or lifelong disabilities, helping them develop mobility strategies, improve functional independence, and access adaptive equipment that supports daily living activities. Rehabilitation programs may involve strength training, assistive device training, environmental modification recommendations, and caregiver education to support long-term independence and safety.

90. Do physical therapists assist with recovery after fractures?

Yes. Physical therapists frequently work with patients recovering from fractures once medical stabilization allows safe movement progression. Rehabilitation focuses on restoring joint mobility, rebuilding strength, improving balance, and helping patients gradually return to normal functional activities. Treatment timelines vary depending on fracture location, surgical involvement, and individual healing rates, requiring careful progression planning to avoid reinjury.

91. Can physical therapists help patients manage arthritis?

Yes. Rehabilitation for arthritis commonly includes joint-protection education, strengthening exercises that support joint stability, flexibility training, and activity-modification strategies designed to reduce pain during daily activities. Therapists also teach pacing techniques that help individuals maintain activity participation while minimizing symptom flare-ups. These approaches aim to preserve mobility and functional independence over the long term.

92. How important is professional accountability in physical therapy?

Professional accountability is essential because therapists are responsible for clinical decision-making that directly affects patient safety and functional outcomes. Accountability includes accurate documentation, adherence to clinical guidelines, ongoing professional education, and ethical treatment practices. Maintaining accountability ensures high-quality care and preserves public trust in the profession.

93. Do physical therapists participate in community education programs?

Yes. Many therapists participate in community education initiatives such as fall-prevention workshops, injury-prevention seminars, workplace ergonomics training, and public health outreach programs focused on maintaining mobility and functional health. These initiatives help increase awareness of rehabilitation services and promote proactive health maintenance across communities.

94. Can physical therapists work in interdisciplinary rehabilitation teams for complex medical cases?

Yes. Physical therapists are integral members of interdisciplinary rehabilitation teams managing complex medical cases involving trauma recovery, neurological injury, multi-system illness, or long-term disability. Collaboration with physicians, occupational therapists, speech-language pathologists, nurses, and social workers ensures coordinated treatment planning that addresses both medical and functional recovery needs.

95. Do physical therapists help patients regain independence after serious illness?

Yes. Physical therapists play a key role in helping patients recover functional independence following serious illnesses such as stroke, severe infections, prolonged hospitalizations, or major surgical procedures. Rehabilitation focuses on rebuilding strength, endurance, balance, and mobility so individuals can safely perform daily activities such as walking, transferring, dressing, and household tasks. Gradual functional progression helps patients transition from medically dependent care toward independent living whenever possible.

96. Can physical therapists work in long-term care facilities?

Yes. Many therapists work in long-term care or skilled nursing facilities where they provide rehabilitation services for residents recovering from surgery, managing chronic conditions, or experiencing mobility decline related to aging. Treatment often focuses on maintaining mobility, preventing functional deterioration, reducing fall risk, and supporting residents' ability to perform daily activities safely within the facility environment.

97. How important is patient safety in physical therapy practice?

Patient safety is a primary responsibility in all rehabilitation settings. Therapists must carefully evaluate medical history, physical tolerance, and environmental risks before initiating treatment activities. Monitoring vital signs, providing appropriate assistance during mobility tasks, and adjusting treatment intensity based on patient response all contribute to safe rehabilitation progression. Safety awareness protects patients from injury while supporting effective recovery.

98. Do physical therapists collaborate with family members or caregivers?

Yes. Collaboration with family members and caregivers is often essential, particularly when patients require assistance at home or are recovering from complex medical conditions. Therapists teach caregivers safe transfer techniques, exercise assistance methods, and mobility-support strategies that help patients continue rehabilitation activities outside clinical sessions. Caregiver education strengthens treatment continuity and improves long-term recovery outcomes.

99. Can physical therapists work in rehabilitation program development?

Yes. Experienced therapists sometimes participate in designing rehabilitation programs within hospitals, outpatient clinics, wellness centers, or community health initiatives. Program development roles may involve creating treatment protocols, designing injury-prevention programs, implementing outcome-tracking systems, and evaluating rehabilitation service effectiveness. These positions combine clinical expertise with organizational planning skills to improve care delivery systems.

100. What personal qualities help someone succeed as a physical therapist over the long term?

Long-term success in physical therapy often depends on a combination of resilience, adaptability, communication skill, and sustained professional curiosity. Therapists who remain open to learning new treatment approaches, adjusting to evolving healthcare systems, and refining time-management strategies tend to maintain stronger career satisfaction. Patience is also essential, as rehabilitation progress is often gradual and requires sustained encouragement of patients who may feel discouraged at various points in recovery. Clinicians who find meaning in helping individuals regain independence, who are comfortable working closely with people throughout extended recovery timelines, and who are willing to adjust practice settings when necessary frequently experience the greatest long-term sustainability in the profession.

101. If I am being completely honest with myself, should

I become a physical therapist — or would another path fit me better?

This profession demands more than interest in exercise or healthcare. It requires comfort with sustained patient interaction, tolerance for documentation responsibilities, physical stamina throughout full clinical days, and the willingness to guide individuals through recovery processes that can be slow and sometimes emotionally complex. Many people are capable of performing the technical tasks required in rehabilitation, but long-term fulfillment depends on whether the daily realities of the work — the pace, productivity expectations, interpersonal demands, and physical activity level — align with who you are and how you prefer to work. If the core activities of teaching movement, coaching recovery, and working closely with patients over time genuinely energize you, the profession may fit well. If those daily demands feel misaligned with your preferences, exploring adjacent healthcare roles that better match your working style may lead to stronger long-term satisfaction.

Chapter 24
Money Map™

Pay Reality, Hidden Costs, and Financial Tradeoffs

Understanding compensation in physical therapy requires looking beyond starting salary figures and examining the full financial landscape of the profession over time. While compensation varies by region, practice setting, and experience level, most physical therapists enter the workforce with doctoral-level education costs that may require careful long-term financial planning. Tuition for Doctor of Physical Therapy programs can represent a significant investment, and prospective students benefit from calculating total projected borrowing, estimated monthly repayment obligations, and expected early-career income before committing to a program. The financial experience of the profession is therefore shaped not only by earnings but also by the relationship between education cost, repayment structure, and long-term earning trajectory.

Entry-level compensation for physical therapists typically falls within a moderate professional salary range compared with other doctoral-level healthcare roles. Earnings often increase gradually over time as clinicians gain experience, move into specialty areas, assume supervisory responsibilities, or transition into leadership roles. Certain settings—such as home health, travel therapy, or geographically underserved regions—may offer higher compensation packages or temporary incentives due to workforce demand, though these roles may involve additional travel, productivity expectations, or variable scheduling requirements. Outpatient settings sometimes include productivity-based compensation models in which earnings are tied partially to patient volume or service delivery targets, making workflow efficiency an important factor in income growth.

Benefits packages can significantly influence total compensation and should be evaluated alongside salary figures. Employer-sponsored health insurance, retirement contributions, continuing education reimbursement, licensure fee coverage, and paid professional development opportunities represent meaningful financial value over time. Some healthcare systems also offer loan repayment assistance programs, sign-on bonuses, or retention incentives designed to attract clinicians to high-demand practice areas. When comparing job offers, evaluating total compensation—including benefits, schedule stability, and long-term advancement opportunities—often provides a clearer financial picture than salary alone.

Hidden costs associated with the profession should also be considered. Continuing education requirements, specialty certification courses, professional association memberships, and licensing fees represent recurring professional expenses throughout a therapist's career. While some employers cover these costs, others may not, making it important for clinicians to understand what financial support is included in employment agreements. Additionally, productivity-driven environments may influence workload intensity, which can indirectly affect long-term career sustainability if compensation structures are not balanced with manageable patient volumes.

Financial growth opportunities do exist within the profession, particularly for therapists who pursue specialty certification, clinical leadership roles, administrative positions, consulting work, or private practice ownership. Clinic ownership or partnership models can provide increased earning potential over time, though they also introduce operational expenses, staffing responsibilities, and business management risks that differ from traditional employment roles. Some clinicians diversify income through teaching, continuing education instruction, ergonomic consulting, or rehabilitation program development, creating multiple revenue streams that expand long-term financial stability.

Ultimately, the financial outlook of physical therapy is best understood as a long-term progression rather than a rapid early-career income surge. Individuals who plan educational financing carefully, select practice settings aligned with both lifestyle and financial goals, and pursue professional advancement opportunities strategically often achieve stable and sustainable earnings over time. Evaluating the profession through this broader financial lens—education investment, compensation growth, benefits, and advancement pathways—allows prospective therapists to make informed decisions about whether the long-term financial structure of the career aligns with their expectations and priorities.

Chapter 25

Pivot Playbook™ — Career Flexibility and Exit Ramps Within Physical Therapy

One of the most valuable features of the physical therapy profession is its structural flexibility. Although many individuals enter the field envisioning a single long-term practice setting, most therapists evolve professionally over time, shifting toward environments, specialties, or hybrid roles that better match their interests, physical capacity, lifestyle priorities, or financial goals. Understanding potential pivot pathways early in a career allows clinicians to make proactive decisions rather than feeling confined to a single role when circumstances change.

The most common pivot occurs between clinical practice settings. A therapist may begin in outpatient orthopedics to build foundational musculoskeletal skills, later transition into inpatient rehabilitation for exposure to complex neurological or post-surgical cases, and eventually move into home health, telehealth, academic teaching, or specialty performance environments. Because the core clinical license remains the same across most settings, many of these transitions require only short periods of mentorship, targeted continuing education, or workplace orientation rather than formal retraining programs. This portability allows therapists to adjust the pace, intensity, and workflow structure of their careers while remaining within the profession.

Specialty development represents another important pivot pathway. Therapists may pursue advanced training or board certification in areas such as orthopedics, neurology, pediatrics, geriatrics, sports rehabilitation, cardiovascular and pulmonary rehabilitation, or women's health. Specialization can increase clinical expertise, expand referral networks, and open opportunities for teaching, mentorship, or leadership roles within rehabilitation organizations. For clinicians who prefer deeper expertise rather than broader generalist practice, specialty certification provides a structured pathway for professional growth.

Leadership and administrative roles offer additional pivot opportunities for therapists seeking reduced direct patient-care intensity later in their careers. Department management, clinical supervision, rehabilitation program coordination, quality improvement leadership, and healthcare operations roles allow experienced clinicians to apply their clinical knowledge at a systems level. These transitions often occur gradually, beginning with mentorship responsibilities, committee participation, or part-time supervisory roles before expanding into full administrative leadership positions.

Entrepreneurial pathways also exist for therapists interested in business ownership or consulting. Private practice clinics, mobile therapy services, performance training centers, ergonomics consulting firms, and workplace injury-prevention programs represent common entrepreneurial models within the profession. While these roles offer increased autonomy and potential income growth, they also introduce responsibilities related to staffing, compliance, marketing, and financial management. Many successful clinician-entrepreneurs build experience as employees first, learning reimbursement systems and operational workflows before launching independent ventures.

Non-clinical pivots provide another dimension of flexibility. Physical therapists may transition into medical device consulting, rehabilitation technology development, insurance utilization review, healthcare policy work, research, academic faculty roles, or professional association leadership. These pathways allow clinicians to remain connected to the field while shifting the nature of their daily work away from direct patient treatment. Such transitions are often supported by advanced education, research involvement, or specialized professional certifications developed over time.

Career pivots are not signs of leaving the profession; they are evidence of how broadly rehabilitation expertise can be applied. Therapists who periodically reassess their workload preferences, professional interests, and long-term lifestyle goals often discover multiple opportunities to reshape their careers while maintaining the professional identity they worked hard to build. Viewing physical therapy as a flexible career platform rather than a single fixed role allows clinicians to design long-term professional trajectories that remain aligned with both personal and professional priorities.

Chapter 26

Before You Apply to School™

What Prospective Physical Therapy Students Should Know First

Before applying to a Doctor of Physical Therapy (DPT) program, prospective students benefit from developing a clear understanding of the profession's daily realities, educational investment, and long-term career structure. Physical therapy is often introduced to students through short observation experiences that highlight patient interaction and rehabilitation success stories, but the full professional picture also includes documentation requirements, productivity expectations in some clinical settings, and the physical stamina required to sustain patient-facing work across long clinical days. Entering the educational pathway with a realistic understanding of these elements helps applicants determine whether the profession aligns with both their interests and their long-term lifestyle expectations.

Academic preparation is an important early consideration. Most DPT programs require completion of prerequisite science coursework, including anatomy, physiology, physics, biology, and statistics, along with competitive academic performance across these subjects. Because admission to many programs is selective, students often strengthen their applications through observation hours in multiple clinical settings, part-time work as rehabilitation technicians or therapy aides, and involvement in healthcare volunteer activities that demonstrate commitment to patient-centered work. Exposure to diverse practice environments—such as hospitals, outpatient clinics, pediatric programs, or neurological rehabilitation settings—helps applicants gain a realistic understanding of how different therapy roles operate day to day.

Financial planning is equally important before applying. The doctoral-level educational pathway represents a multi-year financial commitment, and applicants benefit from estimating tuition costs, living expenses during full-time study, expected borrowing levels, and projected loan repayment obligations after graduation. Comparing these projections with anticipated early-career earnings allows students to make informed decisions about school selection, scholarship opportunities, and geographic employment strategies after graduation. Some students choose programs that offer lower tuition costs or strong clinical placement networks to support early career employment opportunities.

Understanding the structure of clinical education is another key step. DPT programs require extended full-time clinical rotations in multiple settings, which may involve temporary relocation or travel. Preparing for the logistical realities of these placements—housing arrangements, transportation, and schedule flexibility—helps students avoid unexpected challenges during training. Clinical rotations often serve as early employment networking opportunities as well, making professional conduct and engagement during these experiences especially important.

Prospective applicants should also reflect honestly on their personal motivations for entering the profession. Interest in movement science, enjoyment of coaching and teaching others, comfort with sustained patient interaction, and willingness to work in physically active environments are strong indicators of professional alignment. While the profession offers meaningful opportunities to help individuals regain independence and improve quality of life, long-term satisfaction is most likely when individuals choose the career with a clear understanding of both its rewards and its operational demands.

Applying to physical therapy school is not only an academic decision but also a strategic life decision involving financial planning, career expectations, and long-term professional identity. Taking time to research programs carefully, gain meaningful clinical exposure, and evaluate long-term goals before submitting applications allows prospective students to enter the educational pathway with confidence, clarity, and realistic expectations about the journey ahead.

Chapter 27
Terms of Care™

Understanding Compensation, Expectations, and Negotiation

Entering the workforce as a physical therapist involves more than accepting a salary figure. Each employment offer represents a structured agreement that defines workload expectations, compensation structure, productivity targets, scheduling flexibility, professional development support, and long-term advancement potential. Understanding these elements before signing an employment contract helps clinicians avoid misalignment between professional expectations and daily work realities. Many early-career therapists focus primarily on base salary when evaluating offers, yet the broader employment framework often has greater long-term influence on career satisfaction and financial stability.

Compensation structures in physical therapy vary across settings. Some organizations offer fixed salary models, while others include productivity-based compensation systems in which a portion of earnings depends on patient visit volume, billable service targets, or performance-based incentives. Understanding how productivity is calculated—whether through visit counts, relative value units, or service thresholds—is essential before accepting a position. Clinicians should ask how productivity expectations compare with current staff performance, how documentation time is accounted for within productivity models, and whether support staff are available to assist with workflow efficiency. These operational details significantly influence daily workload intensity.

Benefits packages represent another critical component of employment evaluation. Health insurance coverage, retirement contributions, continuing education reimbursement, licensure fee support, paid professional development time, and paid time off all contribute to the total value of an employment offer. Some employers also provide sign-on bonuses, relocation assistance, or student loan repayment incentives designed to attract clinicians to high-demand regions. When comparing multiple job opportunities, evaluating the full compensation package rather than salary alone provides a more accurate understanding of financial value over time.

Scheduling expectations and workload structure should also be reviewed carefully. Some outpatient clinics operate with tightly scheduled patient appointments that allow limited buffer time between sessions, while hospital-based positions may involve weekend rotations or holiday coverage requirements. Home health roles may provide flexible scheduling but require travel time management and geographic productivity planning. Understanding how schedules are structured, how cancellations are handled, and how productivity expectations adjust during seasonal fluctuations can help clinicians anticipate realistic daily workflows before beginning a new role.

Negotiation is often underutilized by early-career clinicians who assume employment terms are fixed. While not all components of an offer are negotiable, many employers are open to discussing continuing education funding, professional conference support, mentorship opportunities, schedule preferences, or gradual productivity ramp-up periods for new graduates. Approaching negotiation as a collaborative discussion rather than a confrontation often leads to mutually beneficial adjustments that support long-term professional success.

Clarifying expectations during the hiring process also helps prevent misunderstandings later. Questions about mentorship availability, onboarding structure, documentation training, and opportunities for specialty development provide insight into how organizations support clinician growth. Employers that invest in structured onboarding programs, continuing education pathways, and leadership development opportunities often create environments where clinicians remain longer and advance professionally.

The goal of reviewing Terms of Care™ is not simply to secure the highest starting salary but to ensure the full employment agreement aligns with professional goals, preferred workload structure, and long-term career trajectory. When clinicians evaluate compensation, expectations, productivity models, and professional development opportunities together, they gain a clearer understanding of whether a role supports both immediate employment needs and long-term career sustainability.

Chapter 28

The 90-Day Pathway™

The first ninety days in a new physical therapy role often shape long-term confidence, workflow efficiency, and professional satisfaction. This early period is not simply about proving competence; it is about learning how the organization functions, understanding documentation expectations, developing communication patterns with interdisciplinary teams, and gradually building clinical rhythm within the specific demands of the workplace. Approaching the first three months as a structured adaptation phase rather than an immediate performance test helps new clinicians transition more smoothly into long-term success.

During the first thirty days, the primary focus should be orientation and observation. Learning electronic documentation systems (gl), understanding productivity measurement methods, reviewing organizational treatment protocols, and observing experienced clinicians can accelerate early competence. Many new therapists benefit from asking detailed workflow questions during this phase, including how experienced staff manage documentation time, organize treatment sessions efficiently, and coordinate communication with physicians or case managers. Establishing mentorship relationships early creates a reliable source of guidance as clinical independence increases.

Days thirty through sixty often involve expanding clinical independence while continuing skill refinement. Caseloads typically increase gradually, allowing clinicians to develop time-management strategies and documentation routines that support sustainable productivity. This phase often includes identifying personal efficiency techniques—such as documenting portions of sessions in real time, preparing treatment plans in advance, or organizing therapy materials before sessions begin—that reduce administrative backlog. Building consistent patient communication routines during this period also strengthens therapeutic relationships and improves session flow.

During days sixty through ninety, clinicians often reach a point of operational familiarity, allowing attention to shift toward long-term professional development. At this stage, therapists may begin identifying continuing education priorities, exploring specialty interests, or seeking opportunities to participate in departmental initiatives such as quality improvement projects or mentorship activities. Understanding long-term growth pathways early in employment helps align daily work with future career direction.

Across the full ninety-day period, self-monitoring of workload sustainability is important. Adjusting pacing strategies, maintaining physical conditioning, and establishing routines that support recovery from physically active workdays help prevent early-career fatigue. Open communication with supervisors about onboarding needs, mentorship availability, and workload progression also contributes to smoother adaptation and stronger early professional performance.

The 90-Day Pathway™ is not designed as a rigid timeline but as a structured transition framework. Clinicians who treat the first three months as a learning phase—focused on workflow mastery, professional relationship development, and gradual productivity growth—often build stronger long-term confidence and stability in their roles. Thoughtful onboarding experiences frequently set the foundation for both early-career success and long-term professional sustainability.

Chapter 29

Professional Development Roadmap™ — Planning Your Physical Therapy Career Trajectory

Career growth in physical therapy rarely occurs by accident. Clinicians who plan intentionally for skill development, specialty exploration, and leadership opportunities often experience greater professional satisfaction and long-term stability. A structured professional development roadmap helps therapists move beyond entry-level clinical practice toward expanded expertise, advanced responsibility, and diversified career pathways over time.

Year 1 — Clinical Foundation and Workflow Mastery

The first year of practice focuses primarily on building clinical confidence, refining evaluation skills, and developing efficient documentation and time-management habits. Early-career therapists benefit from seeking mentorship, attending foundational continuing education courses, and observing experienced clinicians to strengthen clinical reasoning. Establishing strong patient communication habits during this phase creates a foundation for long-term professional success.

Years 2–5 — Skill Expansion and Specialty Exploration

After gaining baseline clinical experience, therapists often begin exploring specialty interests such as orthopedics, neurology, pediatrics, sports rehabilitation, geriatrics, or cardiopulmonary care. Continuing education becomes more targeted, and some clinicians begin accumulating the clinical experience required for specialty certification pathways. Participation in professional organizations, conference attendance, and mentorship of students or new graduates often begins during this period as professional identity strengthens.

Years 5–10 — Leadership Development and Advanced Expertise

Mid-career therapists frequently move into supervisory, mentorship, or program coordination roles. Some pursue board certification in specialty areas, while others explore administrative leadership positions, teaching opportunities, or research collaboration. Developing leadership, communication, and operational planning skills during this phase can open doors to department management or academic faculty roles.

Years 10+ — Career Diversification and Strategic Pivot Opportunities

Later career stages often involve diversification into advanced leadership, consulting, private practice ownership, academic teaching, healthcare administration, or rehabilitation program development. Some clinicians transition into hybrid roles that combine clinical practice with management, education, or consulting responsibilities. These career pivots allow therapists to continue contributing their expertise while adjusting workload intensity or professional focus to match evolving life priorities.

Professional development is not a linear process, and timelines vary widely across individuals. However, clinicians who periodically reassess their interests, pursue targeted education, and remain open to evolving career opportunities often build careers that remain both sustainable and professionally rewarding over decades of practice.

Chapter 30

Technology and Innovation™ — Navigating the Digital Transformation of Rehabilitation

Technology is rapidly reshaping rehabilitation practice, influencing how physical therapists document care, track outcomes, communicate with patients, and deliver treatment services across both in-person and remote environments. Understanding how digital systems integrate into daily clinical workflows helps therapists remain efficient, adaptable, and prepared for evolving healthcare delivery models.

Electronic health record (EHR) systems form the operational backbone of most clinical environments. Therapists use these platforms to document evaluations, treatment sessions, progress reports, and discharge summaries while communicating with interdisciplinary care teams. Developing efficient documentation habits within these systems significantly improves workflow sustainability, particularly in environments where productivity expectations (gl) are closely tied to documentation completion.

Wearable technology and digital movement-monitoring tools are increasingly used to measure rehabilitation progress objectively. Motion-tracking devices, smart braces, and activity-monitoring applications provide clinicians with real-time data on patient movement patterns, adherence to exercise programs, and functional activity levels outside therapy sessions. These tools allow therapists to adjust treatment plans using measurable performance indicators rather than relying solely on subjective reporting.

Telehealth platforms represent another expanding dimension of rehabilitation care. Virtual therapy sessions allow clinicians to guide exercises, monitor patient technique, provide education, and assess functional mobility remotely. Telehealth services expand access to care for individuals in rural areas or those with transportation limitations while offering clinicians additional scheduling flexibility. Effective telehealth practice requires strong verbal instruction skills, careful visual observation, and patient education strategies that ensure safe independent exercise performance.

Assistive technology innovations are also improving rehabilitation outcomes. Advanced prosthetics, robotic-assisted gait training systems, exoskeleton mobility devices, and adaptive mobility equipment continue to expand the possibilities of functional recovery for individuals with complex mobility impairments. Therapists working in advanced rehabilitation environments may collaborate with biomedical engineers and rehabilitation technology specialists to integrate these tools into treatment programs.

Artificial intelligence and predictive analytics are beginning to influence rehabilitation planning as well. Outcome-tracking systems that analyze patient progress data can help identify treatment effectiveness trends, predict recovery timelines, and support evidence-based decision-making. While these technologies are still evolving, clinicians who remain informed about digital rehabilitation tools position themselves to adapt more easily as healthcare systems continue integrating data-driven care models.

Technology does not replace clinical judgment; it enhances it. Therapists who learn to integrate digital tools into patient care while maintaining strong hands-on clinical reasoning skills are better prepared to navigate the modern rehabilitation landscape. As healthcare continues shifting toward hybrid care delivery models combining in-person and virtual services, technological fluency will become an increasingly valuable professional competency within the field of physical therapy.

Chapter 31

Alignment Check & Reflection™

Choosing a healthcare career is not only about capability; it is about long-term alignment between the demands of the profession and the realities of how you prefer to live and work. Physical therapy offers meaningful opportunities to help individuals regain independence, improve mobility, and return to daily activities that matter to them. At the same time, the profession involves productivity expectations in many settings, consistent documentation responsibilities, physically active workdays, and sustained patient interaction across extended recovery timelines. Reflecting honestly on how these elements fit your preferences is essential before committing to the path.

Consider how you respond to work that requires repeated patient interaction throughout the day. Some individuals find deep satisfaction in coaching, teaching, and guiding patients through incremental progress over weeks or months, while others prefer faster-paced clinical decision-making environments with shorter patient encounters. Reflecting on whether long-term therapeutic relationships energize you or drain you can provide insight into whether rehabilitation practice aligns with your working style.

Physical stamina and daily workflow structure also deserve consideration. Many therapists spend large portions of the day standing, demonstrating exercises, assisting mobility tasks, and maintaining sustained attention across multiple patient sessions. Individuals who enjoy physically active work environments often find this energizing, while those who prefer primarily desk-based roles may experience the demands differently over time. Long-term sustainability often depends on how well the daily physical rhythm of the job matches personal comfort and endurance levels.

Financial structure is another important element of alignment. The educational investment required for doctoral-level training should be evaluated alongside long-term compensation expectations, benefits packages, and career advancement opportunities. Some clinicians find the financial structure of the profession well-aligned with their long-term goals, while others discover that adjacent healthcare roles offer compensation models better suited to their priorities. Honest evaluation of education cost, earning trajectory, and lifestyle goals helps clarify whether the financial framework of the profession fits long-term planning.

Finally, consider how adaptable the profession feels to you. Physical therapy offers multiple career pathways—clinical specialization, leadership roles, teaching opportunities, consulting work, and entrepreneurial ventures—that allow professionals to reshape their careers over time. For individuals who value career flexibility and enjoy developing new professional directions throughout their working lives, this adaptability can be a major advantage.

Alignment is not determined by whether you can succeed in the profession; it is determined by whether the daily experience of the work fits who you are over the long term. Taking time to reflect on your motivations, preferences, and long-range goals allows you to approach the decision with clarity, ensuring that the path you choose is not only achievable but sustainable.

Chapter 32

Student Success Stories™ — Six Journeys Into the Physical Therapy Profession

Story 1 — The Career-Changer Who Found His Second Start

Henry had already lived an entire career before physical therapy ever entered his life. For nearly fifteen years he worked in warehouse logistics, supervising shipping teams, managing schedules, and handling operational deadlines that rarely paused for holidays or family events. The work paid the bills, but it never felt like something he intended to do long term. Like many people, he stayed because stability felt safer than uncertainty. Over time, however, the physical demands of repetitive lifting, combined with a nagging shoulder injury that refused to fully resolve, pushed him into the healthcare system as a patient.

His first exposure to rehabilitation came after orthopedic surgery (gl) recommended months of physical therapy. At first, he expected therapy to be a short series of exercises designed simply to restore strength. Instead, he found himself working with a therapist who explained not only the mechanics of recovery but also the biomechanics of how his job tasks had contributed to the injury in the first place. The sessions gradually shifted from simple strengthening exercises to movement retraining, posture education, and long-term injury prevention planning. For the first time, Henry saw healthcare not only as treatment but as education.

During those appointments, he noticed something that stayed with him: the therapist spent most of each session coaching, teaching, and encouraging rather than simply performing procedures. Patients left the clinic walking a little easier, standing a little straighter, or moving with a little more confidence than when they arrived. The idea that a profession could combine science, coaching, and visible daily progress sparked a curiosity Henry had not felt about work in years.

The thought of returning to school in his mid-thirties initially felt unrealistic. He had a mortgage, a young daughter, and responsibilities that did not pause for academic exploration. Yet the idea kept returning. After researching the profession more deeply, he realized that becoming a physical therapist would require completing prerequisite science courses (gl), gaining observation hours (gl), and eventually applying to a Doctor of Physical Therapy program. The path looked long, but it also looked purposeful in a way his previous career never had.

Henry began cautiously, enrolling in evening anatomy and physiology (gl) courses at a local community college while continuing to work full time. The first semester felt overwhelming. Balancing late-night studying with early-morning work shifts required discipline he had not used in years. There were moments when he questioned whether the transition was realistic, especially when assignments piled up or financial stress increased. What helped most was seeing incremental progress—passing each course, completing each prerequisite, and gradually building academic confidence he had once believed he lacked.

Observation hours at a rehabilitation clinic confirmed that he was moving in the right direction. Watching therapists manage patient caseloads, document treatment sessions, and collaborate with physicians (gl) and occupational therapists (gl) showed him that the profession required both clinical knowledge and operational organization. The environment was busy, sometimes fast-paced, but the sense of purpose he felt while assisting patients with simple mobility tasks convinced him the transition was worth the effort.

Admission into a DPT program did not arrive easily. Henry applied twice before receiving an acceptance letter, using the intervening year to strengthen his application, improve prerequisite grades, and continue building observation experience. When acceptance finally came, the decision to step away from full-time employment and commit to graduate study represented one of the most significant financial and personal risks he had ever taken. His family adjusted budgets, relocated temporarily for clinical rotations, and relied on long-term planning to navigate the transition.

The academic program challenged him in ways he had not anticipated. Courses in kinesiology (gl), neurorehabilitation (gl), and clinical reasoning demanded consistent preparation, and clinical rotations required adapting to multiple healthcare settings within short periods. Yet his prior work experience unexpectedly became an advantage. Years spent managing schedules, coordinating teams, and solving logistical problems made time management during clinical training far more manageable than he had expected.

His first full-time clinical placement occurred in an outpatient orthopedic clinic, where he worked under the supervision of an experienced therapist who encouraged gradual independence. Early sessions focused on observing patient evaluations (gl), assisting with exercise instruction, and learning documentation systems. Within weeks, he began conducting portions of treatment sessions independently, gaining confidence as patients responded positively to his coaching style. The moment he guided a patient through a successful return-to-work plan following a workplace injury marked a turning point—he realized he had transitioned fully from patient to clinician.

After graduation and licensure (gl), Henry accepted a position in a community outpatient clinic that served a wide range of patients, from post-surgical recovery cases to individuals managing chronic mobility conditions. The early months were demanding, particularly as he adjusted to productivity expectations and documentation timelines, but the satisfaction of seeing patients regain functional mobility (gl) reinforced his decision daily. Over time, he developed a particular interest in workplace injury prevention programs, eventually collaborating with local employers to design ergonomic (gl) training sessions aimed at reducing repeat injuries.

Today, Henry often speaks with prospective students who are considering career changes later in life. His message is consistent: entering the profession does not require a perfectly linear educational path. What it requires is a willingness to commit to the learning process, realistic financial planning, and a clear understanding of why the work matters personally. His journey demonstrates that alignment is not always discovered early; sometimes it is found after years spent in roles that simply help people recognize what they truly want their work to accomplish.

Story 2 — The First-Generation Student Who Built a New Path

Elena grew up in a household where college was discussed more as an aspiration than an expectation. Her parents worked multiple jobs to support the family, and while education was always encouraged, the logistics of navigating applications, financial aid, and career planning often felt unfamiliar territory. During high school, Elena excelled academically but had only a general idea that she wanted to work in healthcare. What she did not yet know was which role would allow her to combine her interest in science, her natural patience with people, and her desire to help individuals regain independence after injury.

Her introduction to rehabilitation occurred when her grandmother suffered a stroke (gl) that required months of recovery. Elena watched therapists work with her grandmother repeatedly on mobility training, balance exercises, and speech coordination. Progress was slow but visible, and the patience required during each session left a strong impression. She noticed that therapists celebrated small improvements—a stronger grip, a steadier step, a longer standing time—as meaningful milestones rather than minor achievements. That perspective shifted her understanding of healthcare from crisis treatment to long-term recovery support.

Entering college as a first-generation student brought challenges she had not anticipated. Navigating academic advising, prerequisite planning, and financial aid applications required learning systems that many of her classmates already understood through family guidance. During her first year, she balanced part-time employment with full course loads, occasionally questioning whether the path toward a Doctor of Physical Therapy program was realistic given the cost and length of training. What helped sustain her motivation was consistent exposure to the profession through volunteer hours at a rehabilitation hospital, where she assisted therapy aides with preparing treatment areas and escorting patients between departments.

These volunteer experiences revealed the complexity of rehabilitation work. Therapists evaluated functional mobility (gl), assessed range of motion (gl), and developed individualized treatment plans that adapted as patients improved. Elena realized that physical therapy required far more than exercise instruction; it involved clinical reasoning, patient education, and collaboration with interdisciplinary (gl) healthcare teams. Observing these interactions strengthened her commitment to pursuing the field despite the financial and academic challenges ahead.

Applying to graduate programs required persistence. Elena spent months preparing for standardized admissions exams, completing observation hour requirements, and refining application essays that described both her academic goals and her personal motivation for entering the profession. When she received her first acceptance letter, the moment felt less like a finish line and more like confirmation that years of preparation had opened a door she once believed might remain closed.

Graduate training presented a new level of academic intensity. Courses in neuroanatomy, pathology (gl), and therapeutic exercise (gl) required extensive study time, and clinical rotations placed her in unfamiliar healthcare environments that demanded rapid adaptation. During her first inpatient rehabilitation rotation, she worked with patients recovering from spinal cord injuries (gl), traumatic brain injuries (gl), and major orthopedic surgeries (gl). The emotional weight of these cases was sometimes difficult, particularly when patients faced long recovery timelines, but she also witnessed remarkable resilience that reinforced the value of the work.

Elena's final clinical placement occurred in a community outpatient clinic serving a diverse patient population. There she learned to balance patient scheduling demands, documentation requirements (gl), and treatment progression planning while maintaining the communication skills necessary to keep patients motivated through repetitive rehabilitation exercises. By the end of the rotation, she recognized that professional confidence develops gradually through consistent patient interaction rather than arriving suddenly at graduation.

After licensure (gl), Elena accepted a position in a hospital-based outpatient program where mentorship opportunities were built into the onboarding process. Working alongside experienced therapists allowed her to refine treatment planning strategies, improve documentation efficiency, and begin exploring specialty interests in neurological rehabilitation. Over time, she became particularly interested in stroke recovery programs, eventually helping develop group-based therapy sessions designed to improve patient engagement and peer support during long-term rehabilitation.

Today, Elena often returns to local colleges to speak with students who are considering healthcare careers but feel uncertain about navigating the process as first-generation applicants. Her message is simple: lack of familiarity with the system does not mean lack of capability. With consistent planning, mentorship, and willingness to seek guidance, pathways that once appear complicated gradually become manageable. Her journey reflects not only professional achievement but also the broader impact of representation—showing future students that careers in rehabilitation are accessible even when the starting point feels unfamiliar.

Story 3 — The ICU Nurse Who Wanted to Help Patients Recover, Not Just Survive

Daniel had spent eight years working as an intensive care unit nurse, a role defined by urgency, rapid decision-making, and the constant awareness that small clinical changes could mean the difference between stabilization and decline. He was skilled, respected by colleagues, and deeply committed to patient care. Yet over time, he noticed something that gradually reshaped how he viewed his professional future: many of the patients he helped save in the ICU disappeared from his life the moment they transferred out of the unit. He rarely saw what recovery looked like beyond stabilization.

The turning point came when a patient he had cared for following a severe motor vehicle accident returned months later to visit the ICU staff. The patient walked in slowly, supported by a cane, accompanied by a physical therapist who had guided months of rehabilitation. Watching that interaction made Daniel realize that the recovery phase—the long, patient process of helping individuals rebuild strength, mobility, and independence—was a part of healthcare he had never experienced directly as a clinician. The idea of participating in that phase began to take hold.

At first, the thought of leaving nursing felt risky. He had already invested years in education, built clinical experience, and developed financial stability. Transitioning into another healthcare profession would require returning to school, completing prerequisite coursework, and applying to a Doctor of Physical Therapy program. The commitment was significant, but the desire to work more directly in functional recovery continued to grow.

Daniel began researching the overlap between critical care recovery and rehabilitation medicine. He learned that patients who survive extended ICU stays often require structured rehabilitation programs to regain muscle strength lost during prolonged immobilization (gl). This connection between acute care survival and long-term functional recovery helped him see how his previous clinical experience could translate meaningfully into a rehabilitation career. Rather than abandoning his nursing background, he realized he could build upon it.

Completing the transition required careful planning. Daniel enrolled in the additional prerequisite science courses necessary for DPT program admission while continuing part-time nursing shifts to maintain income. Balancing coursework with clinical responsibilities tested his endurance, yet the clarity of his professional goal helped sustain motivation through the demanding schedule. Observation hours in both inpatient rehabilitation and outpatient clinics reinforced that the pace of rehabilitation work differed from critical care but carried its own intellectual and physical challenges.

Graduate training proved academically demanding but professionally rewarding. Courses in musculoskeletal evaluation (gl), neuromotor rehabilitation (gl), and therapeutic intervention planning (gl) expanded his understanding of how movement recovery is structured across different patient populations. During clinical rotations, he found that his prior experience communicating with critically ill patients and families gave him confidence when working with individuals facing long recovery timelines. He was comfortable explaining treatment plans, setting realistic expectations, and supporting patients emotionally during difficult stages of rehabilitation.

Daniel's first professional position after licensure (gl) was in an inpatient rehabilitation hospital specializing in post-surgical and neurological recovery. There he worked with patients transitioning from acute care settings, helping them relearn mobility skills, balance strategies, and functional transfers (gl) necessary for returning home safely. The work was physically demanding and required careful coordination with interdisciplinary (gl) teams, including occupational therapists, speech-language pathologists, and physicians, but it also provided the long-term patient continuity he had been seeking.

One of the most meaningful aspects of the role was witnessing full recovery arcs. Patients he met during their earliest rehabilitation stages often returned months later walking independently, resuming work activities, or participating in family routines they once feared might be permanently lost. That continuity—seeing individuals move from severe impairment to restored independence—reinforced Daniel's decision to change careers.

Today, he occasionally mentors nurses who express curiosity about rehabilitation careers, emphasizing that career transitions within healthcare are more common than many professionals realize. Skills developed in one discipline often transfer effectively to another, particularly when communication, clinical observation, and patient education are involved. His journey illustrates that professional growth sometimes involves moving closer to the aspect of healthcare work that feels most personally meaningful, even when doing so requires stepping outside an established role.

Story 4 — The Athlete Who Wanted to Keep Others in the Game

Jordan spent most of adolescence on a soccer field. Practices before school, strength sessions in the afternoon, and weekend tournaments shaped a routine that revolved around competition and performance. For years, injuries were treated as temporary obstacles—sprained ankles, muscle strains, and occasional overuse injuries that required brief physical therapy visits before returning to play. What began as routine treatment gradually became something more influential. Jordan noticed that the therapists guiding rehabilitation were not simply helping athletes recover; they were teaching them how to understand their own bodies.

During a senior-year season, a significant knee injury changed everything. Instead of returning to the field after a few weeks, Jordan entered a months-long rehabilitation process that required structured strengthening, neuromuscular training (gl), and careful progression through functional movement milestones. The recovery period was frustrating, but it also provided an extended view of how rehabilitation programs were designed. Therapists tracked range of motion (gl), monitored gait (gl) mechanics, and adjusted exercises based on measurable progress rather than arbitrary timelines. The experience sparked an interest that gradually evolved into a career decision.

Entering college, Jordan initially planned to study sports management, assuming the path would remain connected to athletics. However, volunteering in the campus athletic training facility provided exposure to injury prevention programs, post-surgical rehabilitation, and performance recovery protocols that closely resembled the therapy experience following the knee injury. Conversations with clinicians introduced the possibility of pursuing physical therapy as a profession, combining scientific study with the opportunity to help athletes and active individuals return to performance safely.

Academic preparation required shifting coursework toward prerequisite sciences (gl), including anatomy, physiology (gl), and physics (gl), while continuing part-time work assisting in the athletic department. Balancing demanding science courses with volunteer commitments proved challenging, yet the direct connection between coursework and future professional goals strengthened motivation. Observation hours in outpatient sports rehabilitation clinics confirmed that the profession extended far beyond professional athletics; therapists worked with individuals of all ages seeking to return to recreational activity, work duties, or daily functional movement.

Graduate training introduced Jordan to a wider spectrum of rehabilitation practice. Clinical rotations included inpatient neurological rehabilitation, outpatient orthopedic clinics, and community-based wellness programs, each demonstrating different aspects of patient care. While sports rehabilitation remained the long-term interest, exposure to diverse patient populations reinforced the importance of developing broad foundational clinical reasoning skills before specializing.

The transition into professional practice began in a general outpatient orthopedic clinic where patient cases ranged from post-surgical recovery to chronic joint pain management. Although the patient population was broader than originally expected, the setting provided valuable experience refining evaluation techniques, treatment progression planning, and patient education strategies. Over time, Jordan pursued continuing education courses focused on sports performance rehabilitation and injury prevention programming, gradually building a referral network that included local athletic organizations and recreational sports leagues.

Eventually, an opportunity emerged to join a multidisciplinary sports performance center where therapists collaborated with strength coaches, athletic trainers, and physicians to support athletes across training and recovery cycles. The role combined injury rehabilitation, movement screening programs, and performance optimization services designed to reduce reinjury risk. Working with athletes ranging from high school competitors to adult recreational players reinforced the realization that rehabilitation is not solely about returning to sport—it is about helping individuals sustain active lifestyles over the long term.

Jordan now mentors student volunteers who assist in the clinic, often sharing the perspective that injuries can become unexpected entry points into meaningful careers. The experience of rehabilitation as a patient provided firsthand understanding of the emotional challenges individuals face during recovery, shaping a treatment approach built on both technical expertise and empathy. What began as a setback on the playing field ultimately became the foundation for a career dedicated to helping others remain active, resilient, and engaged in the activities they value most.

Story 5 — The Single Parent Who Built a Long-Term Career Step by Step

Tanya did not begin her professional journey with a long-range academic plan. After high school, she entered the workforce quickly, taking administrative and customer-service positions that allowed her to support herself financially. When she became a parent in her early twenties, stability became the primary priority. Career exploration often took a back seat to work schedules, childcare logistics, and the daily demands of building a household on a single income.

Her introduction to physical therapy came unexpectedly when her son required rehabilitation following a sports-related injury. Attending therapy appointments exposed her to the clinical environment in a way she had never experienced before. She watched therapists guide patients through strengthening exercises, mobility training, and balance interventions (gl), often explaining the purpose behind each activity in clear, accessible language. What stood out most was how consistently therapists combined technical knowledge with encouragement, helping patients remain motivated even during slow recovery periods.

Curiosity gradually turned into career interest. Tanya began researching rehabilitation professions, initially assuming that entering healthcare would require immediate enrollment in a lengthy academic program that was financially unrealistic. Instead, she discovered entry-level support roles such as rehabilitation technician (gl) positions that allowed individuals to work within therapy environments while gaining exposure to clinical workflows. Applying for one of these roles marked the first step toward a career transition she had not previously considered possible.

Working as a rehabilitation technician provided daily exposure to treatment sessions, patient documentation systems, and interdisciplinary (gl) team communication. While the position focused primarily on preparing treatment spaces, assisting with equipment setup, and supporting patient flow, the experience helped her understand the operational rhythm of rehabilitation clinics. Conversations with therapists revealed multiple educational pathways, including the possibility of completing prerequisite coursework gradually while continuing to work.

Balancing employment, parenting responsibilities, and part-time coursework required long-term planning. Tanya enrolled in evening community college classes to complete foundational science prerequisites (gl), often studying late at night after her child was asleep. Progress was slower than that of traditional full-time students, yet each completed course represented tangible movement toward a long-term goal. Financial planning, scholarship applications, and careful scheduling allowed her to continue advancing without abandoning employment entirely.

Acceptance into a Doctor of Physical Therapy program represented a significant milestone, but it also required restructuring family routines and financial priorities. Extended clinical rotations (gl) sometimes required temporary schedule adjustments and additional childcare coordination, yet the support network she had built over time helped sustain the transition. The determination that had carried her through years of balancing responsibilities became one of her strongest professional assets during graduate training.

After licensure (gl), Tanya accepted a position in a community outpatient clinic that emphasized mentorship for new graduates. The early months of practice required adjustment to productivity expectations, documentation timelines, and the physical pace of clinical workdays, but her years of prior clinic experience as a technician made the environment feel familiar. Over time, she developed a strong interest in working with patients managing chronic musculoskeletal (gl) conditions, focusing on long-term functional improvement rather than short-term symptom relief.

Today, Tanya often encourages individuals who believe they have “missed the window” for healthcare careers to reconsider that assumption. Her path into the profession was not linear or accelerated; it was built gradually through small, consistent steps that accumulated into a long-term career transformation. Her experience illustrates that professional timing varies widely, and with structured planning, persistence, and incremental progress, significant career changes remain achievable even when life responsibilities make the journey more complex.

Story 6 — The Military Medic Who Transitioned to Civilian Rehabilitation

Andre spent most of his early adult life in structured environments where decisions were made quickly and precision mattered. As a military medic, he developed skills in emergency stabilization, trauma response, and field-based medical assessment. The work required resilience, discipline, and the ability to function effectively under pressure, but it also exposed him to the long-term consequences of physical injuries sustained during training and deployment. While emergency care focused on immediate survival, he often wondered what happened to individuals months or years after those initial interventions.

Near the end of his military service, Andre participated in a rehabilitation program designed to help injured service members regain mobility and functional strength. Observing physical therapists work with patients recovering from orthopedic surgeries (gl), amputations (gl), and neurological injuries (gl) introduced him to a different dimension of healthcare—one focused not on crisis response but on long-term restoration of independence. The process was slower, less dramatic than emergency medicine, yet equally impactful in shaping patients' lives.

Transitioning from military service to civilian career planning required translating prior experience into new professional pathways. Andre learned that many of his medical training hours could support admission into prerequisite science coursework (gl), allowing him to accelerate the academic preparation needed for a Doctor of Physical Therapy program. Veterans' education benefits also provided financial assistance that made the educational transition more manageable.

Returning to the classroom after years of military service presented an adjustment period. Academic pacing differed from operational environments, and learning advanced subjects such as kinesiology (gl), pathology, and evidence-based rehabilitation (gl) required sustained study habits. However, the discipline developed during military training helped him maintain structured routines, allowing him to progress steadily through coursework and clinical training requirements.

Clinical rotations introduced Andre to diverse patient populations, including individuals recovering from joint replacement surgeries (gl), stroke rehabilitation (gl), and chronic mobility limitations. His prior experience working in high-stress medical environments proved beneficial when communicating with patients facing uncertain recovery timelines. He was comfortable providing clear instructions, setting realistic expectations, and maintaining composure during complex treatment situations.

After completing licensure (gl), Andre accepted a position in an inpatient rehabilitation hospital where many patients were transitioning from acute medical care to functional recovery programs. The setting required coordination with interdisciplinary (gl) teams, including occupational therapists, speech-language pathologists, nurses, and physicians, to develop comprehensive rehabilitation plans. The structured teamwork environment felt familiar, echoing the coordinated systems he had experienced during military service.

Over time, Andre developed a professional interest in working with veterans recovering from service-related injuries, eventually participating in community outreach programs that connected former service members with rehabilitation resources. Helping individuals navigate recovery after significant injuries allowed him to continue serving a population he deeply understood while building a long-term civilian healthcare career.

Today, he frequently advises transitioning service members that skills developed in military healthcare roles often translate effectively into civilian rehabilitation professions. Clinical discipline, teamwork experience, and adaptability provide strong foundations for success in structured healthcare environments. His career demonstrates how prior service experience can evolve into a new professional identity, one that continues the mission of helping others regain independence and functional strength long after initial injuries occur.

Chapter 33

Work Settings Deep Comparison™

Understanding Where Physical Therapists Work — and How Daily Life Changes by Setting

One of the most important decisions physical therapists make throughout their careers is not simply what specialty to pursue, but which practice setting best aligns with their preferred workflow, energy patterns, and long-term professional goals. Although licensure allows therapists to work across many environments, the daily experience of the job can vary dramatically depending on where care is delivered. Understanding these differences helps clinicians select positions that match both their clinical interests and lifestyle preferences.

Outpatient Orthopedic Clinics

Outpatient orthopedic clinics represent one of the most common practice settings for physical therapists. These environments primarily treat musculoskeletal (gl) conditions such as joint injuries, post-surgical rehabilitation cases, chronic pain syndromes (gl), and sports-related injuries. Therapists in outpatient clinics typically manage scheduled appointments throughout the day, working with multiple patients in structured treatment sessions. Productivity expectations may be closely tied to visit volume, making efficient documentation and time management essential skills. Clinicians who enjoy active patient coaching, structured scheduling, and long-term treatment relationships often find outpatient practice rewarding. However, the pace can be demanding in high-volume clinics where documentation time must be balanced carefully with patient care responsibilities.

Inpatient Rehabilitation Hospitals

Inpatient rehabilitation facilities focus on individuals recovering from major medical events such as stroke (gl), spinal cord injury, traumatic brain injury, or complex surgical procedures. Therapists in these settings often work with patients for longer treatment sessions, concentrating on mobility training, functional independence development, and discharge planning. Interdisciplinary (gl) collaboration is a central component of daily workflow, with therapists participating in team rounds alongside physicians, nurses, occupational therapists, and speech-language pathologists. Clinicians who enjoy collaborative care environments and the opportunity to witness significant functional recovery over concentrated rehabilitation periods often find inpatient practice highly meaningful.

Skilled Nursing Facilities (SNFs)

Skilled nursing facilities provide rehabilitation services for individuals who require continued recovery support following hospitalization but may not need intensive inpatient rehabilitation programs. Therapists in SNFs often work with older adults managing post-surgical recovery, mobility decline, or chronic health conditions affecting functional independence. Treatment sessions may emphasize balance training (gl), fall prevention strategies, and activities of daily living (gl) mobility support. Workflow structures vary widely across facilities, and productivity expectations may influence daily scheduling intensity. Therapists who value working with geriatric populations and supporting gradual functional improvement often find this setting professionally fulfilling.

Home Health Practice

Home health physical therapy involves delivering rehabilitation services directly within patients' homes. This setting allows therapists to evaluate functional mobility (gl) within real-world environments, identifying safety risks such as uneven flooring, limited accessibility, or environmental obstacles affecting recovery. Scheduling often involves independent time management, with therapists traveling between patient locations throughout the day. While the autonomy of home health practice appeals to many clinicians, travel logistics, documentation timelines, and geographic caseload planning require strong organizational skills. Therapists who prefer independence and flexible scheduling often find home health roles particularly attractive.

Sports Performance and Specialty Rehabilitation Centers

Sports rehabilitation and performance centers focus on injury recovery, movement optimization, and performance enhancement for athletic populations ranging from youth athletes to professional competitors. Therapists in these settings often collaborate with strength coaches, athletic trainers, and sports physicians to design rehabilitation programs that support safe return-to-sport progression. Movement screening, injury prevention programming, and performance conditioning may complement traditional rehabilitation interventions. Clinicians with strong interests in athletics, biomechanics, and performance science often pursue these specialized practice environments.

Selecting a work setting is not a permanent decision; many therapists transition between environments as their careers evolve. Early-career clinicians may begin in general outpatient practice to build foundational experience before moving into specialty roles, leadership positions, or hybrid clinical-administrative pathways. Understanding the operational differences between practice settings allows therapists to make informed decisions about where their professional strengths, preferred workflow intensity, and long-term career goals align most effectively.

Chapter 34

First Five Years Strategy™

Surviving, Stabilizing, and Specializing

The first five years of a physical therapy career often determine long-term professional trajectory more than any other period. Early decisions about work setting, mentorship opportunities, skill development, and specialty exploration shape not only clinical confidence but also long-term career sustainability. Approaching these initial years with a structured development strategy helps therapists avoid common early-career burnout patterns while building a strong professional foundation.

Year 1 — Stabilization and Workflow Mastery

The first professional year focuses primarily on adaptation. New therapists learn documentation systems, productivity expectations, scheduling patterns, and the operational rhythm of clinical environments. During this phase, the most important goal is consistency rather than speed. Developing reliable evaluation routines, treatment progression frameworks, and patient communication strategies builds confidence that gradually improves efficiency. Seeking mentorship from experienced clinicians during this period significantly accelerates learning and helps prevent avoidable early-career stress.

Years 2–3 — Competence Expansion and Confidence Building

As operational familiarity increases, therapists begin refining clinical reasoning skills and expanding treatment approaches across broader patient populations. Continuing education courses often become more targeted, focusing on specific clinical interests such as orthopedic rehabilitation, neurological recovery, or sports injury management. Therapists in this stage frequently begin identifying which patient populations and clinical challenges energize them most, providing early signals that guide future specialization decisions.

Years 3–4 — Strategic Skill Positioning

Midway through the first five-year period, therapists often begin positioning themselves for long-term professional growth. Some pursue specialty certification pathways (gl), while others explore leadership opportunities such as student mentorship, clinical education roles, or department-based quality improvement initiatives. Developing strong professional networks during this phase also increases access to future career opportunities, particularly in competitive specialty practice areas.

Year 5 — Specialization or Strategic Pivot

By the fifth year of practice, many therapists reach a stage where foundational clinical competence is well established. At this point, some clinicians pursue advanced specialization tracks, leadership development roles, or transitions into new practice settings that better match evolving career interests. Others begin exploring hybrid roles that combine patient care with administrative, teaching, or consulting responsibilities. The decisions made at this stage often shape the next decade of professional direction.

The first five years are not about achieving perfection; they are about building sustainable systems of practice. Therapists who intentionally focus on mentorship, continuing education, and gradual skill expansion during this period often experience greater long-term career stability. Viewing early practice as a structured development phase rather than a performance race allows clinicians to grow steadily while maintaining professional resilience.

Chapter 35

First Five Years Strategy™

Skill, Income, Leverage, and Professional Positioning

The first five years of a physical therapy career shape long-term professional trajectory more than most clinicians initially realize. During this early period, therapists develop core clinical habits, establish professional networks, determine specialty interests, and build the operational knowledge that influences future income growth and career flexibility. Approaching these years with an intentional strategy helps clinicians accelerate both skill development and long-term opportunity creation.

Year 1 — Foundation and Workflow Mastery

The primary objective during the first professional year is establishing consistency in evaluation procedures, treatment planning routines, and documentation systems. New therapists often focus heavily on clinical decision-making, but workflow efficiency—scheduling management, documentation pacing, and patient communication systems—is equally important. Developing strong daily operational habits early reduces stress and prevents administrative backlog patterns that can follow clinicians for years if not corrected.

Years 2–3 — Skill Expansion and Specialty Exploration

As foundational clinical routines stabilize, therapists begin identifying clinical populations or specialty areas that align with professional interests. Continuing education courses, mentorship relationships, and exposure to diverse patient cases help clinicians determine whether they prefer orthopedic rehabilitation, neurological (gl) recovery, sports performance, geriatric mobility programs, or other specialized practice areas. Exploring specialty pathways early allows clinicians to begin building expertise that differentiates them within the workforce.

Years 3–4 — Income Awareness and Role Positioning

By the third or fourth year, therapists typically gain a clearer understanding of compensation structures, productivity expectations, and advancement opportunities across different work settings. This stage often involves evaluating whether current employment environments provide both financial growth potential and sustainable workload structures. Some clinicians begin exploring leadership roles, program development opportunities, or specialty certification pathways (gl) that expand long-term earning potential.

Year 5 — Strategic Career Direction Decisions

Approaching the fifth year of practice, therapists often reach a decision point regarding long-term career direction. Some pursue advanced specialty certifications, clinical residency programs, or leadership development pathways. Others begin exploring entrepreneurial opportunities such as private practice ownership, consulting services, or hybrid roles combining clinical care with teaching or administrative responsibilities. By this stage, clinicians who have intentionally tracked professional interests and skill development patterns are often positioned to make more confident long-term career decisions.

Building Professional Leverage Early

Professional leverage develops through a combination of clinical competence, specialty expertise, strong professional relationships, and reputation for reliability within healthcare teams. Therapists who maintain mentorship connections, participate in professional associations, and consistently pursue skill development often discover that opportunities for advancement appear more readily than for those who rely solely on time-in-position progression.

The first five years do not determine the entire career, but they strongly influence future flexibility and growth potential. Clinicians who approach this period as a strategic development phase—rather than simply a time of employment experience—often build professional foundations that support decades of career mobility, financial growth, and sustained clinical confidence.

Chapter 36

Twenty-Year Career Architecture™

Designing Longevity in a Physically Demanding Profession

Physical therapy is a profession built on movement, and the same is true of the careers within it. The clinicians who remain satisfied and sustainable over twenty or more years rarely follow a single static path. Instead, they periodically adjust clinical intensity, diversify responsibilities, expand expertise, and redesign how they contribute to patient care as their experience grows. Viewing a physical therapy career as a long-term architecture rather than a fixed job helps clinicians intentionally plan for longevity.

Years 1–5 — Foundation and Skill Acceleration

The early years of practice focus on mastering evaluation techniques, treatment progression planning, documentation efficiency, and interdisciplinary (gl) communication. These years establish the clinical instincts that support later specialization and leadership opportunities. Therapists who invest heavily in continuing education, mentorship relationships, and exposure to multiple patient populations during this period often develop broader clinical confidence that supports future flexibility.

Years 5–10 — Specialization and Professional Identity Formation

Mid-career clinicians frequently begin defining their professional identities more clearly, selecting specialty focus areas such as orthopedics, neurological rehabilitation, pediatrics, sports performance, or geriatric rehabilitation. Some pursue advanced certification pathways (gl), while others begin mentoring students, supervising clinical rotations, or leading small departmental initiatives. This stage often marks the transition from generalist practice toward recognized expertise.

Years 10–15 — Leadership, Teaching, or Hybrid Roles

As experience accumulates, many therapists expand their responsibilities beyond full-time clinical care. Opportunities may include department leadership roles, clinical education coordination, consulting work, program development, or participation in research initiatives. Hybrid positions that combine patient care with administrative or educational responsibilities allow clinicians to maintain clinical involvement while reducing the physical intensity of daily treatment schedules.

Years 15–20+ — Strategic Diversification and Sustainability Planning

Later career stages often emphasize sustainability and long-term professional contribution. Some clinicians transition into executive leadership, academic faculty positions, private practice ownership, or healthcare operations consulting. Others reduce clinical caseload intensity while focusing on mentorship, specialty consultation, or program development roles. The goal during this period is not withdrawal from the profession but strategic adaptation that allows continued engagement without excessive physical strain.

A twenty-year perspective changes how career decisions are made early on. Instead of asking only, "Where should I work now?" clinicians begin asking, "What experiences will give me the flexibility I want ten years from today?" Those who periodically reassess their interests, energy levels, and professional goals often build careers that remain both productive and personally sustainable over decades of practice.

Chapter 37

Professional Associations & Certification Pathways™

Building Credibility, Expertise, and Professional Reach

Professional growth in physical therapy is supported not only by clinical experience but also by engagement with professional associations, continuing education networks, and specialty certification pathways. Participation in these structures allows therapists to remain current with evolving clinical research, expand professional networks, and demonstrate advanced expertise within specific areas of rehabilitation practice. Over time, involvement in professional organizations often opens doors to leadership opportunities, teaching roles, and collaborative research initiatives that extend professional impact beyond daily clinical work.

Professional associations serve as central hubs for education, advocacy, and practice standards. Many therapists join national and regional professional organizations early in their careers to access continuing education courses, clinical practice guidelines, and professional networking opportunities. These organizations frequently host conferences where clinicians share emerging treatment approaches, research findings, and rehabilitation innovations. Attendance at these events allows therapists to exchange ideas with peers, explore specialty interests, and remain informed about regulatory changes affecting the profession.

Certification pathways represent another important dimension of professional development. After accumulating required clinical experience hours, therapists may pursue specialty certifications in areas such as orthopedic rehabilitation, neurological rehabilitation, pediatric care, geriatric rehabilitation, sports rehabilitation, or cardiopulmonary rehabilitation. Certification programs typically involve structured examination processes (gl), clinical case documentation (gl), and continuing education requirements designed to validate advanced competency within the specialty area. While certification is not required for most clinical positions, it often enhances professional credibility, supports career advancement, and may expand referral opportunities within specialized practice settings.

Professional involvement also strengthens leadership development. Many therapists begin by participating in local association committees, student mentorship programs, or conference planning teams, gradually building organizational experience that can lead to regional or national leadership roles. These experiences allow clinicians to contribute to policy development, workforce advocacy, and professional education initiatives that influence the future direction of rehabilitation practice.

Continuing education remains a lifelong responsibility within the profession. Licensing boards typically require periodic continuing education completion to maintain clinical licensure (gl), ensuring that practitioners remain informed about evolving treatment methods and safety standards. Therapists who approach continuing education strategically—selecting courses aligned with long-term career goals rather than completing random credit requirements—often develop deeper expertise that strengthens professional positioning over time.

Professional associations and certification pathways function as long-term career accelerators rather than short-term resume additions. Clinicians who remain engaged with professional networks, pursue specialty education intentionally, and contribute to organizational initiatives often build reputations that extend beyond individual workplaces. Over time, these connections and credentials create opportunities for leadership, consulting, and advanced clinical practice that shape the trajectory of an entire career.

Chapter 38

Advanced Specialization Tracks™

Orthopedic, Neurological, Pediatric, Sports, Pelvic, and Geriatric Pathways

As physical therapists gain clinical experience, many begin exploring specialty pathways that allow them to focus more deeply on specific patient populations or clinical problem areas. Specialization does not occur immediately after graduation; it typically develops through years of patient exposure, targeted continuing education, mentorship, and eventually formal certification processes. Understanding the major specialization tracks helps clinicians plan long-term professional development strategies that align with their clinical interests.

Orthopedic Rehabilitation

Orthopedic specialization focuses on musculoskeletal (gl) injuries, post-surgical recovery, joint dysfunction, and chronic movement-related pain conditions. Therapists in this track frequently work in outpatient clinics, treating patients recovering from ligament repairs, joint replacements, and overuse injuries. Advanced orthopedic clinicians often develop strong expertise in manual therapy (gl), movement analysis, and functional strengthening progression strategies designed to restore full mobility and prevent reinjury.

Neurological Rehabilitation

Neurological rehabilitation specialists work with patients recovering from stroke (gl), spinal cord injuries (gl), traumatic brain injuries (gl), and neurodegenerative (gl) conditions. Treatment often emphasizes motor control retraining, balance recovery, and functional independence development. These therapists frequently practice in inpatient rehabilitation hospitals, outpatient neurological clinics, or specialized rehabilitation centers where interdisciplinary (gl) collaboration plays a central role in patient care.

Pediatric Rehabilitation

Pediatric physical therapists focus on developmental (gl) movement disorders, congenital (gl) conditions, and childhood injuries affecting mobility and functional growth. Treatment programs often involve close collaboration with families, educators, and pediatric healthcare teams to support long-term developmental progress. Clinicians in this track typically work in pediatric hospitals, school-based therapy programs, or specialized outpatient pediatric clinics.

Sports Rehabilitation

Sports rehabilitation specialists focus on injury recovery, performance conditioning, and return-to-sport progression planning for athletic populations. Therapists in this field frequently collaborate with athletic trainers, strength coaches, and sports physicians to develop rehabilitation programs that integrate performance training principles with injury prevention strategies. Work environments may include sports medicine clinics, performance training centers, or collegiate and professional athletic programs.

Pelvic Health Rehabilitation

Pelvic health specialization addresses conditions affecting pelvic floor (gl) function, including post-surgical recovery, pregnancy-related mobility challenges, and chronic pelvic pain disorders. Therapists in this specialty receive additional training to evaluate and treat musculoskeletal and neuromuscular (gl) conditions affecting pelvic stability and functional movement. This area has experienced significant growth as awareness of pelvic health rehabilitation services expands.

Geriatric Rehabilitation

Geriatric specialists focus on mobility preservation, fall prevention, and functional independence among aging populations. Treatment often emphasizes balance training (gl), strength development, and environmental safety planning designed to support long-term independent living. Therapists in this specialty frequently work in skilled nursing facilities, outpatient geriatric clinics, or home health settings serving older adult populations.

Specialization pathways are not rigid career commitments; many therapists develop expertise in more than one area over time or transition between specialties as professional interests evolve. The purpose of specialization is not to narrow career opportunities but to deepen clinical impact within selected areas while maintaining the flexibility that defines rehabilitation practice.

Chapter 39

Compensation Modeling & Lifetime Earnings Pathways™

Understanding Long-Term Financial Growth in Physical Therapy

Evaluating the financial outlook of a physical therapy career requires examining earnings as a long-term progression rather than focusing solely on starting salary. Income growth within the profession typically follows a gradual trajectory influenced by experience level, specialization, geographic location, leadership responsibilities, and entrepreneurial opportunities. Therapists who understand how compensation evolves over time are better positioned to make strategic career decisions that support both financial stability and professional satisfaction.

Early Career Earnings — Establishing the Baseline

During the first several years of practice, compensation is generally tied to entry-level clinical roles where therapists build foundational experience and workflow efficiency. Salary ranges vary by region, healthcare system structure, and practice setting, with some environments offering productivity-based compensation models (gl) that include performance incentives tied to patient volume or service delivery thresholds. While early-career income may feel modest compared with other doctoral-level healthcare professions, the stability of employment and consistent demand for rehabilitation services provide reliable financial footing during the initial stage of career development.

Mid-Career Growth — Experience, Specialization, and Leadership

As therapists accumulate experience and develop specialty expertise, earning potential often increases through supervisory roles, advanced clinical certification pathways (gl), and participation in leadership or program development initiatives. Therapists who pursue specialization in high-demand clinical areas, take on mentorship responsibilities, or transition into departmental leadership roles frequently see incremental compensation growth tied to expanded responsibilities.

Advanced Career Opportunities — Diversification of Income Streams

Later career stages often introduce opportunities for diversified income beyond traditional clinical employment. Private practice ownership, consulting services, ergonomic (gl) program development, continuing education instruction, and clinical research participation represent additional revenue pathways that experienced therapists may explore. Entrepreneurial roles involve greater operational responsibility and financial risk but can significantly expand earning potential over time.

Lifetime Earnings Perspective

When evaluating lifetime earnings, it is important to consider cumulative income across decades of practice rather than short-term salary comparisons. Stable employment demand, consistent salary progression, and the ability to diversify professional roles contribute to long-term financial sustainability. Therapists who combine clinical expertise with leadership development, specialty certification, or entrepreneurial initiatives often create multiple pathways for income growth across their careers.

Financial Planning Considerations

Long-term financial success within the profession is influenced not only by salary growth but also by debt management strategies, retirement planning, continuing education investments, and career positioning decisions made during early practice years. Therapists who actively plan financial milestones—such as loan repayment timelines, savings targets, and investment strategies—often experience greater financial flexibility later in their careers.

Understanding compensation as a dynamic, multi-stage progression allows clinicians to make career decisions that support both professional development and long-term financial goals. Rather than viewing income potential as fixed, therapists who approach career growth strategically often discover multiple opportunities to expand both earnings and professional impact over time.

Chapter 40

Work Setting Comparison — Long-Term Lifestyle Fit™

Choosing Environments That Sustain Career Energy Over Time

Beyond compensation and specialty interest, one of the most significant long-term career decisions for physical therapists involves selecting work environments that align with personal energy patterns, preferred patient interaction styles, and long-term lifestyle priorities. Different practice settings not only influence daily workflow intensity but also shape long-term physical demands, scheduling flexibility, and professional stress levels. Understanding how these factors evolve over time helps therapists design careers that remain sustainable across decades of practice.

High-Volume Outpatient Practice

High-volume outpatient clinics often provide structured daily schedules and predictable work hours, which many clinicians appreciate for long-term planning. However, patient visit density can create sustained pacing demands, particularly in clinics where documentation must be completed within short timeframes. Therapists who thrive in these environments typically develop strong time-management strategies, efficient documentation habits, and structured treatment progression systems that maintain both patient quality of care and workflow sustainability. Over the long term, some clinicians transition into mentorship or supervisory roles within outpatient systems to balance clinical workload intensity with leadership responsibilities.

Hospital-Based Rehabilitation Settings

Hospital-based practice settings, including inpatient rehabilitation units and acute care rehabilitation teams, often provide strong interdisciplinary (gl) collaboration and exposure to complex clinical cases. The pace may fluctuate depending on patient acuity (gl), but many therapists appreciate the team-based care structure and predictable institutional benefits packages. Over time, therapists in hospital systems may transition into program development roles, clinical educator positions, or administrative leadership pathways that allow continued professional engagement while adjusting physical workload demands.

Home Health Practice Models

Home health environments offer significant scheduling autonomy, allowing therapists to structure daily visits independently while traveling between patient homes. This flexibility appeals to clinicians who prefer independent work patterns and geographic variety throughout the day. However, travel time, documentation coordination, and environmental variability require strong organizational systems. Many therapists find that home health roles provide sustainable mid-career options, particularly when flexibility becomes increasingly valuable for balancing personal responsibilities.

Specialty and Performance Environments

Sports rehabilitation centers, pediatric specialty clinics, and neurological rehabilitation programs often attract therapists with strong interests in specific patient populations. These environments can be deeply rewarding but may involve variable scheduling demands, extended treatment sessions, or specialized training requirements. Clinicians who build careers in specialty environments often balance direct patient care with program development, consulting, or teaching roles as their expertise grows.

Career Sustainability Perspective

Long-term career satisfaction rarely depends on a single work setting choice. Many therapists move between environments at different career stages, selecting roles that align with evolving professional interests, family responsibilities, and physical workload preferences. Viewing work setting decisions as adjustable over time rather than permanent commitments allows clinicians to design career paths that remain both professionally meaningful and personally sustainable.

Selecting the right environment at the right career stage often determines whether therapists maintain long-term enthusiasm for the profession. By periodically reassessing workload intensity, scheduling preferences, and clinical interests, clinicians can make strategic transitions that support both professional growth and long-term career longevity.

Chapter 41

First Ten Career Moves™

Strategic Decisions That Shape Long-Term Trajectory

The earliest career decisions physical therapists make often influence professional direction for years to come. While no single path guarantees success, certain early moves consistently strengthen long-term career stability, clinical confidence, and professional flexibility. Viewing the early career period as a sequence of strategic positioning decisions—rather than simply accepting the first available job—helps clinicians build stronger long-term foundations.

1. Choose Mentorship Over Convenience

The first position does not need to be the highest-paying job; it should ideally provide access to experienced clinicians willing to mentor new graduates. Structured onboarding programs, collaborative team environments, and accessible senior clinicians accelerate early clinical reasoning development more effectively than isolated work settings.

2. Master Documentation Early

Efficient documentation habits (gl) significantly reduce long-term administrative stress. Clinicians who develop structured charting systems during their first year often maintain sustainable productivity expectations throughout their careers, preventing the accumulation of after-hours documentation work.

3. Explore Multiple Patient Populations

Gaining exposure to diverse patient populations—orthopedic, neurological, pediatric, and geriatric—helps therapists identify areas of natural interest before committing to specialization. Early diversity of experience often leads to stronger long-term career flexibility.

4. Build Professional Relationships Intentionally

Networking is not limited to conferences or formal events. Daily collaboration with physicians, nurses, occupational therapists, and other interdisciplinary (gl) team members builds professional relationships that often influence future job opportunities and referral pathways.

5. Begin Continuing Education Strategically

Rather than accumulating continuing education credits randomly, therapists benefit from selecting coursework that aligns with long-term career interests. Early targeted education accelerates specialty readiness and strengthens clinical positioning.

6. Learn the Business Side of Healthcare

Understanding reimbursement models (gl), productivity measurement systems, and healthcare operations provides insight into how organizations function. Therapists who understand these systems often make more informed career decisions and are better prepared for leadership opportunities.

7. Track Outcomes and Professional Growth

Maintaining records of clinical outcomes, patient improvement benchmarks, and professional achievements helps therapists demonstrate value when pursuing promotions or specialty roles. Tracking measurable impact strengthens professional portfolios over time.

8. Seek Teaching Opportunities Early

Supervising students, assisting with training sessions, or participating in educational presentations builds communication and leadership skills that become valuable in mid-career advancement pathways.

9. Protect Physical Sustainability

Because physical therapy is a physically active profession, early-career clinicians benefit from developing personal injury-prevention routines, proper body mechanics (gl), and recovery strategies that support long-term career longevity.

10. Reassess Direction Every Two to Three Years

Career satisfaction often depends on periodic reassessment. Evaluating whether current roles support professional growth, lifestyle priorities, and clinical interests allows therapists to pivot strategically before burnout develops.

These early moves are not rigid requirements but guiding principles that help therapists design careers intentionally rather than reactively. Clinicians who approach early career decisions with long-term perspective often create professional pathways that remain adaptable, resilient, and aligned with evolving goals.

Chapter 42
Designing a Sustainable Workweek™

Managing Energy, Productivity, and Recovery

Long-term career sustainability in physical therapy depends not only on clinical skill but also on how therapists structure their workweeks to manage physical energy, cognitive workload, and recovery time. Because many therapy roles involve sustained standing, manual assistance with patient mobility, and continuous patient interaction, small adjustments to scheduling patterns and workflow routines can significantly influence long-term professional endurance.

One of the most effective strategies involves pacing patient scheduling to maintain consistent treatment quality throughout the day. High-density scheduling patterns may increase short-term productivity metrics (gl) but can lead to physical fatigue and reduced documentation accuracy over time. Therapists who collaborate with supervisors to design realistic patient scheduling templates often maintain both clinical performance and long-term job satisfaction more effectively than those who operate at unsustainable pacing levels.

Documentation timing also plays a critical role in workload balance. Completing portions of clinical documentation during treatment sessions—when appropriate—reduces after-hours administrative work and helps maintain clearer clinical recall of patient interactions. Developing efficient charting systems early in practice significantly reduces cumulative workload strain over the course of a career.

Physical recovery practices are equally important. Many therapists incorporate strength maintenance exercises, stretching routines, and ergonomic (gl) work habits to prevent repetitive strain injuries. Proper body mechanics (gl) during patient transfers, lifting assistance, and mobility training sessions not only protect clinicians from injury but also improve treatment efficiency and patient safety.

Cognitive recovery should also be considered. Patient-facing clinical work requires sustained attention, emotional engagement, and rapid clinical decision-making throughout the day. Scheduling short mental breaks between sessions, maintaining hydration, and structuring predictable daily routines can help maintain concentration and reduce decision fatigue (gl) during longer workdays.

Workweek design evolves across career stages. Early-career therapists often focus on maximizing skill development and clinical exposure, while mid-career clinicians may prioritize scheduling flexibility or hybrid roles that combine patient care with teaching, leadership, or consulting responsibilities. Periodically reassessing how weekly schedules align with personal energy patterns allows therapists to make adjustments that support both professional performance and personal well-being.

Sustainable careers are rarely built on intensity alone. They are built on systems that allow clinicians to perform consistently over years and decades. Therapists who intentionally design work routines that balance productivity, physical recovery, and cognitive rest often discover that long-term performance improves when weekly workload structures are aligned with human energy patterns rather than short-term output demands.

Chapter 43

Clinical Competency Ladder™

How Expertise Develops Over Time

Clinical expertise in physical therapy develops gradually through repeated patient encounters, reflection on treatment outcomes, and continuous learning rather than through a single training milestone. Understanding how competency evolves helps therapists set realistic expectations for professional growth and reduces the pressure many early-career clinicians feel to perform at expert levels immediately after graduation.

Stage 1 — Foundational Practitioner (Years 0–2)

During the earliest stage of practice, therapists focus on mastering structured evaluation routines, treatment planning frameworks, and documentation systems. Decision-making often relies heavily on learned protocols and mentorship guidance. Confidence grows as clinicians encounter a wider range of patient presentations and begin recognizing common patterns of recovery progression.

Stage 2 — Developing Clinician (Years 2–5)

As experience accumulates, therapists begin adjusting treatment approaches more independently, applying clinical reasoning to modify interventions based on patient response rather than strictly following standardized protocols. Workflow efficiency improves, and clinicians often start identifying specialty interests that guide continuing education choices.

Stage 3 — Advanced Practitioner (Years 5–10)

Clinicians in this stage typically demonstrate strong pattern recognition (gl), efficient evaluation processes, and the ability to manage complex patient cases with reduced supervision. Many begin mentoring students or new graduates, contributing to program development initiatives, or pursuing specialty certification pathways (gl) that validate advanced expertise.

Stage 4 — Expert Clinician (Years 10+)

Expert practitioners combine deep clinical knowledge with intuitive decision-making developed through years of patient interaction. They often serve as clinical educators, consultants, department leaders, or specialty program developers while continuing patient care roles. Expertise at this stage frequently includes the ability to manage unusual or complex rehabilitation cases and guide interdisciplinary (gl) teams in developing comprehensive treatment strategies.

Clinical competency does not progress at identical speeds for every therapist, nor does advancement occur automatically with time alone. Growth is accelerated by mentorship engagement, targeted continuing education, reflective practice habits, and exposure to diverse patient populations.

Therapists who actively invest in learning throughout their careers often find that expertise develops naturally as experience accumulates.

Understanding the competency ladder helps clinicians maintain perspective during challenging early-career periods. Expertise is not expected immediately; it is built through consistent practice, ongoing education, and the gradual accumulation of clinical insight over years of professional experience.

Chapter 44

Career Flexibility Matrix™

How Physical Therapists Adapt Roles Across a Lifetime

One of the defining advantages of the physical therapy profession is its long-term adaptability. While many healthcare careers involve narrowly defined scopes of practice, physical therapists often move between clinical environments, specialty populations, leadership roles, and hybrid professional responsibilities as their interests and life priorities evolve. Understanding how career flexibility functions over time allows clinicians to design professional pathways that remain dynamic rather than fixed.

Clinical Environment Mobility

Licensed therapists can transition across outpatient clinics, inpatient rehabilitation hospitals, skilled nursing facilities, home health programs, sports performance centers, and specialty rehabilitation environments with relatively limited retraining. This environmental mobility allows clinicians to adjust workload intensity, patient population focus, or scheduling preferences as career stages change. For example, early-career therapists may seek high-volume clinical environments to accelerate skill development, while mid-career clinicians sometimes move into specialty or home health roles that offer different pacing structures.

Specialty Diversification

Many therapists develop expertise in more than one clinical specialty across their careers. A clinician who begins in orthopedic rehabilitation may later expand into sports performance training, neurological rehabilitation, or geriatric mobility programs through continuing education and targeted clinical experience. Specialty diversification increases long-term professional flexibility, particularly when healthcare workforce demands shift over time.

Leadership and Administrative Pathways

Career flexibility also includes transitions into supervisory, management, or healthcare operations roles. Therapists who develop leadership skills, participate in quality improvement initiatives, or manage clinical teams often find opportunities to influence care delivery systems beyond individual patient sessions. Administrative roles can provide long-term career sustainability by reducing the physical intensity associated with full-time patient care.

Educational and Consulting Opportunities

Experienced clinicians frequently move into teaching, clinical education coordination, continuing education instruction, or consulting roles within rehabilitation programs. These pathways allow therapists to share expertise while expanding professional influence beyond a single workplace. Educational roles often combine part-time clinical practice with academic or instructional responsibilities, creating hybrid career models that evolve with experience.

Entrepreneurial Pathways

Some therapists pursue private practice ownership, performance training businesses, rehabilitation consulting services, or ergonomic (gl) workplace injury-prevention programs. Entrepreneurial roles provide increased autonomy and income potential but also introduce responsibilities related to business management, staffing, and regulatory compliance. Clinicians who explore entrepreneurship typically benefit from developing operational knowledge before launching independent ventures.

Career Stage Adaptation

Career flexibility becomes particularly important over decades of practice. Early-career clinicians may prioritize skill acquisition and clinical exposure, mid-career professionals often pursue specialization or leadership roles, and later-career therapists frequently transition toward mentorship, consulting, or hybrid roles that maintain professional engagement while reducing physical workload demands. Viewing career progression as an adaptive system rather than a linear ladder allows therapists to maintain long-term professional relevance and satisfaction.

The flexibility inherent in physical therapy careers means that no single role defines the entire professional journey.

Clinicians who remain open to evolving responsibilities, new learning opportunities, and strategic role adjustments often build careers that remain resilient across changing healthcare environments and personal life stages.

Chapter 45
Interdisciplinary Teamwork in Rehabilitation Practice™

How Collaborative Care Shapes Patient Outcomes

Rehabilitation rarely occurs in isolation. Physical therapists function as part of interdisciplinary (gl) healthcare teams that coordinate treatment planning, discharge preparation, and long-term patient recovery strategies. Understanding how collaborative care operates within different clinical environments allows therapists to work more effectively with colleagues while improving patient outcomes across the continuum of care.

In inpatient rehabilitation settings, teamwork is often highly structured. Physical therapists collaborate daily with occupational therapists, speech-language pathologists, nurses, physicians, case managers, and social workers to coordinate treatment priorities and discharge planning. Each discipline contributes a specialized perspective—mobility training, activities of daily living (gl) development, communication recovery, medical stabilization, and social resource planning—forming a comprehensive rehabilitation strategy. Therapists who actively participate in team rounds and treatment planning discussions often develop stronger clinical insight because they understand how multiple care components interact to influence recovery.

Outpatient environments also depend heavily on interdisciplinary communication, though collaboration may occur less formally. Physical therapists frequently communicate with referring physicians, orthopedic surgeons, pain management specialists, and athletic trainers to provide treatment updates and coordinate return-to-activity timelines. Clear documentation, timely progress reports, and direct communication when treatment goals change help maintain continuity of care across healthcare providers.

In home health settings, interdisciplinary coordination often involves communication across geographic distances. Therapists may collaborate remotely with nursing teams, occupational therapists, and case managers through electronic documentation systems and scheduled care coordination meetings. Because therapists observe patients in their home environments, they often provide valuable insights regarding environmental safety risks, caregiver support needs, and functional mobility (gl) challenges that influence long-term recovery planning.

Effective teamwork requires more than technical communication skills. It also involves understanding the scope of practice (gl) of each discipline, respecting professional expertise, and recognizing when collaborative consultation improves patient outcomes. Therapists who actively seek input from colleagues often identify treatment opportunities that might not be apparent from a single professional perspective.

Interdisciplinary collaboration also supports clinician development. Exposure to the treatment approaches of other healthcare professionals expands clinical reasoning and encourages therapists to consider broader dimensions of patient care beyond isolated mobility goals. Learning how occupational therapists address daily functional tasks, how speech-language pathologists manage communication recovery, or how case managers coordinate discharge resources provides therapists with a more complete understanding of rehabilitation systems.

Healthcare delivery continues moving toward team-based care models, making collaborative skills increasingly valuable. Therapists who communicate clearly, document effectively, and participate actively in interdisciplinary planning often become central contributors to rehabilitation teams. Over time, these collaborative habits strengthen both patient outcomes and professional relationships, reinforcing the shared goal that defines rehabilitation practice: restoring independence through coordinated care.

Chapter 46

Common Early-Career Mistakes Physical Therapists Make™

Lessons That Accelerate Professional Growth

Early-career physical therapists often enter the profession highly motivated, well trained academically, and eager to perform at the highest possible level. Yet the transition from structured academic training to full clinical responsibility introduces operational realities that are not always emphasized during school. Understanding common early-career mistakes allows new clinicians to accelerate learning curves, reduce unnecessary stress, and build sustainable practice habits more quickly.

Trying to Work at Maximum Speed Too Early

Many new therapists feel pressure to match the efficiency of experienced clinicians within the first months of practice. Attempting to move too quickly before developing structured evaluation routines and documentation workflows often leads to errors, missed clinical details, or after-hours charting backlogs. Early practice should prioritize consistency and accuracy rather than speed. Efficiency develops naturally as treatment planning frameworks and patient communication routines become familiar.

Over-Relying on Protocols Without Clinical Adaptation

Clinical protocols provide valuable guidance, but every patient responds differently to rehabilitation interventions. Early-career clinicians sometimes hesitate to adjust treatment progressions when patient responses deviate from expected timelines. Developing clinical reasoning skills involves learning when to modify exercise intensity, pacing, or treatment strategies based on observed outcomes rather than strictly following standardized plans.

Underestimating Documentation Complexity

Documentation requirements (gl) often feel more demanding than expected during the first professional year. Delaying documentation completion until the end of the day frequently leads to incomplete notes, time pressure, or extended work hours. Integrating documentation tasks into daily workflow—completing portions of notes during or immediately after sessions—helps maintain both compliance and work-life balance.

Avoiding Questions to Appear Independent

New clinicians sometimes hesitate to seek mentorship guidance because they worry it may signal lack of confidence. In reality, early consultation with experienced therapists often prevents treatment errors, improves efficiency, and strengthens professional relationships. Asking questions is a sign of professional responsibility, not weakness, particularly during the first years of independent practice.

Neglecting Personal Physical Sustainability

Because therapy work involves lifting assistance, transfer training (gl), and sustained standing, failing to maintain proper body mechanics (gl) and personal conditioning routines can lead to early musculoskeletal (gl) strain. Therapists who apply the same injury-prevention strategies they teach patients—strength training, mobility exercises, and ergonomic positioning—often maintain long-term physical resilience more effectively.

Focusing Only on Clinical Skills While Ignoring Systems Knowledge

Understanding scheduling systems, reimbursement structures, productivity expectations, and operational workflows is just as important as clinical competence. Therapists who learn how healthcare systems function early in their careers often make more strategic career decisions and navigate workplace expectations more effectively.

Early-career mistakes are not signs of professional failure; they are predictable learning milestones. Clinicians who approach the first years of practice with openness to feedback, willingness to refine systems, and commitment to continuous learning typically progress rapidly toward professional confidence. Over time, these early lessons form the foundation for sustainable expertise and long-term career satisfaction.

Chapter 47

Burnout, Sustainability, and Career Longevity™

Protecting Energy in a Helping Profession

Physical therapy is a profession built around helping others regain movement, independence, and confidence, yet the same commitment to patient care that makes the work meaningful can also create cumulative strain if workload intensity, productivity expectations, and physical demands are not balanced with sustainable work practices. Understanding how burnout develops—and how it can be prevented—helps therapists design careers that remain both fulfilling and durable over time.

Burnout rarely appears suddenly. It often develops gradually through repeated cycles of high patient volume, documentation pressure, limited recovery time between workdays, and emotional fatigue associated with caring for patients experiencing pain, disability, or slow recovery progress. Early warning signs may include persistent exhaustion, decreased enthusiasm for patient interactions, difficulty maintaining concentration during treatment planning, or a growing sense that work demands consistently exceed available time and energy resources.

One of the most effective burnout-prevention strategies involves aligning workload expectations with realistic scheduling capacity. Therapists who proactively discuss patient scheduling patterns, documentation timelines, and productivity metrics with supervisors often identify opportunities to adjust workflow structures before chronic overload develops. Small operational changes—such as balanced appointment spacing, protected documentation time, or structured mentorship support for new clinicians—can significantly reduce long-term stress accumulation.

Physical sustainability also plays a central role. The profession requires sustained standing, demonstration of exercises, and occasional lifting assistance during mobility training sessions. Maintaining personal strength conditioning routines, applying proper body mechanics (gl), and incorporating recovery practices outside work hours help reduce the risk of cumulative musculoskeletal (gl) strain that can contribute to long-term fatigue.

Career flexibility provides another important protection against burnout. Therapists who periodically reassess work settings, specialty focus, and workload intensity often discover opportunities to transition into environments better aligned with evolving professional interests or life-stage priorities. Movement between outpatient clinics, inpatient rehabilitation settings, home health roles, teaching positions, or leadership pathways allows clinicians to adjust career structure without leaving the profession entirely.

Professional purpose also influences resilience. Clinicians who maintain clear connections to why they entered rehabilitation practice—helping patients regain independence, return to meaningful activities, or recover functional mobility (gl)—often find that sustained purpose buffers against periods of operational stress. Mentorship, participation in professional associations, and engagement in continuing education activities can reinforce this sense of professional identity and long-term commitment.

Career longevity in physical therapy is rarely determined by technical skill alone; it is shaped by how well clinicians design systems that protect both their physical energy and emotional engagement over time. Therapists who actively manage workload sustainability, maintain professional flexibility, and invest in recovery practices often find that meaningful careers in rehabilitation can extend comfortably across decades of practice.

Chapter 48

Mentorship, Teaching, and Giving Back™

Strengthening the Profession Through Shared Knowledge

Every generation of physical therapists benefits from the clinicians who choose to teach, mentor, and guide those entering the profession. While early career stages focus primarily on skill development and clinical confidence, many therapists eventually discover that helping students and newer clinicians grow becomes one of the most professionally rewarding aspects of long-term practice. Mentorship not only strengthens individual careers; it improves the profession as a whole by preserving institutional knowledge, clinical insight, and professional standards across generations.

Mentorship often begins informally. Experienced therapists answer clinical questions from new graduates, demonstrate evaluation techniques, and share workflow strategies that help newer clinicians navigate documentation systems, scheduling structures, and treatment planning challenges. Over time, these informal interactions often evolve into structured mentorship roles such as supervising clinical rotations, serving as clinical instructors, or participating in onboarding programs for newly hired therapists.

Teaching opportunities extend beyond direct supervision. Many therapists contribute to continuing education courses, conference presentations, or in-service training sessions within healthcare organizations. These educational roles allow clinicians to share specialty expertise, introduce emerging rehabilitation techniques, and support professional development within their workplaces. Teaching also reinforces the instructor's own clinical knowledge, as explaining treatment concepts often deepens personal understanding of underlying clinical reasoning processes.

Academic pathways provide another avenue for professional contribution. Some clinicians transition into part-time or full-time faculty roles within physical therapy education programs, combining clinical experience with classroom instruction and research involvement. Academic roles often allow therapists to shape curriculum development, mentor future clinicians, and participate in research initiatives that advance rehabilitation practice.

Mentorship also strengthens professional networks. Therapists who engage actively in mentoring relationships often build connections across healthcare organizations, educational institutions, and professional associations. These relationships frequently lead to collaborative opportunities, leadership roles, and program development initiatives that extend professional impact beyond individual patient care.

Giving back to the profession is not limited to formal teaching roles. Participating in student career panels, volunteering with community health programs, or mentoring early-career clinicians within the workplace all contribute to the professional ecosystem that supports future therapists. These activities help ensure that new clinicians enter the field with realistic expectations, strong foundational skills, and access to experienced guidance.

Over the course of a career, the role of a therapist often evolves from learner to teacher. Clinicians who choose to invest time in mentorship and education frequently discover that the process enriches their own professional experience while strengthening the resilience and quality of the rehabilitation workforce as a whole.

Chapter 49

Final Alignment Synthesis™

Is This Career Right for You?

Physical therapy is a profession built on the belief that movement restores possibility. Every day, therapists work with individuals who are relearning how to walk, return to work, regain independence after injury, or participate again in activities that define their quality of life. The work is meaningful, visible, and often deeply rewarding. At the same time, the profession requires sustained physical activity, careful documentation, productivity expectations, and long-term patient engagement that can span weeks or months of recovery. Deciding whether the career fits you involves evaluating both the purpose of the work and the operational realities that shape daily practice.

Consider how you respond to professions centered on coaching and teaching rather than performing procedures alone. Much of rehabilitation involves guiding patients through repeated practice, encouraging consistency, and helping individuals remain motivated even when progress feels slow.

Individuals who enjoy mentoring, problem-solving, and observing gradual improvement often find strong alignment with the rhythm of rehabilitation practice.

Reflect also on the physical nature of the work. Physical therapists spend significant portions of the day standing, demonstrating exercises, assisting mobility tasks, and maintaining continuous patient interaction. For individuals who prefer active, movement-oriented work environments, this aspect of the profession can be energizing. Those who prefer primarily desk-based roles may experience the physical pace differently over time, making it important to evaluate long-term comfort with the activity level required.

Financial structure represents another important alignment factor. Entering the profession typically requires doctoral-level education, and prospective clinicians benefit from evaluating educational investment alongside long-term compensation trajectories, benefits structures, and advancement opportunities. Long-term financial satisfaction often depends on how well educational costs, expected earnings, and lifestyle priorities align.

Career flexibility is a significant advantage within the profession. Therapists can move between outpatient clinics, hospital rehabilitation programs, home health services, specialty rehabilitation environments, leadership roles, teaching positions, or consulting pathways as their interests evolve. This adaptability allows clinicians to redesign their careers over time rather than remaining fixed in a single professional role.

Ultimately, the most important question is not whether you are capable of becoming a physical therapist; it is whether the daily experience of the profession matches how you want to spend your working life. Careers feel sustainable when the tasks required each day align with personal energy patterns, interests, and long-term goals. If guiding recovery, teaching movement, and supporting long-term functional independence resonate with your strengths and motivations, physical therapy can offer a career that remains both stable and meaningful across decades of practice.

Chapter 50

Closing Reflection — The Long View of a Career in Physical Therapy

Every healthcare career looks different from the inside than it does from the outside. From a distance, physical therapy can appear to be primarily about exercise instruction, rehabilitation equipment, and scheduled treatment sessions. In practice, the profession is far broader. It involves long-term patient relationships, detailed clinical reasoning, interdisciplinary (gl) collaboration, and the responsibility of guiding individuals through recovery processes that often require patience, persistence, and trust.

Throughout this book, you have explored the realities of the profession across multiple dimensions: daily clinical workflows, education requirements, compensation structures, work-setting variations, specialization pathways, and the long-term evolution of physical therapy careers. These elements exist not to persuade you toward the profession, but to provide clarity so that any decision you make is informed rather than assumed. Healthcare careers influence financial planning, lifestyle structure, physical workload, and long-term professional identity, making thoughtful career selection one of the most important decisions many individuals will make.

The most sustainable careers are rarely chosen based solely on job availability or external expectations. They are built on alignment between personal strengths, preferred work environments, long-term lifestyle goals, and the daily activities required by the role. For some readers, the responsibilities of rehabilitation practice—teaching movement, supporting recovery, and maintaining physically active clinical workdays—will feel energizing and purposeful. For others, the demands may highlight a preference for different healthcare roles that better match their desired workflow patterns. Both outcomes represent success, because clarity prevents years spent pursuing paths that do not truly fit.

Physical therapy remains an essential profession within modern healthcare systems, addressing mobility limitations, injury recovery, chronic pain management, and functional independence across the lifespan. As populations age and the demand for rehabilitation services continues to grow, the need for skilled therapists will remain strong. For individuals whose interests align with movement science, patient education, and long-term functional recovery, the profession offers the opportunity to build careers that combine stability with meaningful daily impact.

The purpose of this guide has never been to make the decision for you. Its purpose is to help you see the profession clearly—its rewards, its demands, and its long-term possibilities—so that whatever path you choose is one that reflects both informed understanding and intentional direction.

Chapter 51

Looking Forward — Your Next Step

If you have reached this point in the book, you have already done something many individuals never take the time to do: you have examined a career not only through the lens of job descriptions and salary ranges, but through the realities of daily work, long-term sustainability, and personal alignment. That perspective alone places you ahead of many career decisions that are made based only on surface-level information.

Your next step does not need to be dramatic. For some readers, it may involve scheduling observation hours (gl) in a local rehabilitation clinic to experience the environment firsthand. For others, it may mean speaking with practicing therapists about their daily routines, exploring prerequisite coursework requirements, or mapping the financial planning steps necessary for entering a Doctor of Physical Therapy program. Even small exploratory actions—attending an informational session, volunteering in a rehabilitation setting, or reviewing program admission timelines—begin transforming curiosity into actionable planning.

If you are already pursuing the educational pathway, consider using the insights from this guide to evaluate clinical rotation (gl) opportunities carefully. Exposure to multiple work settings early in training allows you to identify which environments best match your energy patterns, clinical interests, and long-term lifestyle priorities. The earlier alignment becomes visible, the more intentionally you can shape your career trajectory.

For clinicians already practicing in related healthcare roles, the path forward may involve evaluating how existing clinical experience translates into rehabilitation careers or adjacent specialty opportunities. Many professionals discover that previous healthcare experience provides transferable skills that shorten learning curves during career transitions.

Regardless of where you stand in the decision process, remember that career development rarely follows a single straight line. Most successful professionals adjust direction multiple times as they gain new information, encounter new opportunities, and refine their understanding of what type of work feels most meaningful. What matters most is not choosing perfectly at the first step, but continuing to make informed adjustments as your experience grows.

Physical therapy offers a pathway that blends science, movement, education, and long-term patient relationships. Whether you ultimately choose this profession or another healthcare path, the process of evaluating alignment—understanding how work, lifestyle, and purpose intersect—will serve you throughout every stage of your professional life.

Chapter 52
Professional Associations and Continuing Growth™

Staying Current in a Rapidly Evolving Field

Healthcare professions evolve continuously as new research findings, treatment technologies, and care delivery models emerge. For physical therapists, maintaining professional growth requires engagement beyond initial licensure through continuing education, professional associations, and lifelong learning practices that keep clinical knowledge current and practice standards aligned with emerging evidence.

Professional associations play a central role in this process. Organizations such as national and state physical therapy associations provide continuing education courses, clinical practice updates, specialty certification pathways (gl), legislative advocacy resources, and networking opportunities that support long-term professional development. Membership often gives clinicians access to journals, research summaries, clinical guidelines, and conferences where emerging rehabilitation strategies are introduced and discussed.

Continuing education requirements also ensure that therapists remain current with evolving clinical standards. Many states require licensed therapists to complete a defined number of continuing education hours within renewal cycles, encouraging clinicians to update treatment knowledge, refine evaluation techniques, and remain informed about regulatory changes that affect practice. Clinicians who select continuing education topics strategically—based on specialty interests or emerging patient population needs—often develop expertise that expands both career opportunities and treatment effectiveness.

Networking through professional associations provides additional long-term benefits. Conferences, workshops, and professional forums allow therapists to connect with peers, learn from experienced clinicians, and discover emerging career pathways within rehabilitation practice. These professional relationships frequently lead to mentorship opportunities, collaborative research projects, leadership roles, or specialty program development initiatives.

Leadership involvement within professional organizations represents another avenue for career growth. Serving on committees, contributing to advocacy efforts, or participating in policy discussions allows clinicians to influence healthcare systems that shape rehabilitation practice. Therapists who engage in leadership roles often gain broader insight into workforce trends, reimbursement policies (gl), and healthcare delivery models that influence long-term career strategy.

Professional growth does not occur automatically with time; it develops through intentional engagement with learning opportunities and professional communities. Therapists who consistently invest in continuing education, association participation, and knowledge-sharing activities often find that their careers remain dynamic, relevant, and intellectually stimulating across decades of practice.

Chapter 53

Technology in Rehabilitation Practice™

AI, Robotics, Digital Therapy, and the Future of Physical Therapy

Technology is reshaping nearly every aspect of healthcare delivery, and rehabilitation practice is no exception. While the core of physical therapy remains grounded in human interaction, clinical reasoning, and therapeutic movement training, emerging technologies are expanding how therapists evaluate patients, monitor recovery progress, and deliver treatment across both in-person and remote environments. Understanding these technological shifts helps clinicians prepare for a profession that will increasingly blend hands-on care with digital support systems.

Wearable technology represents one of the most rapidly expanding tools in rehabilitation. Motion-tracking sensors, activity-monitoring devices, and wearable strength and balance measurement systems allow therapists to collect objective movement data outside the clinic environment. These tools enable clinicians to monitor gait patterns, joint mobility trends, exercise adherence, and functional activity levels across days or weeks rather than relying solely on in-session observation. As wearable accuracy improves, therapists gain access to longitudinal (gl) data that provides deeper insight into recovery progression and treatment effectiveness.

Remote rehabilitation platforms are also transforming access to care. Tele-rehabilitation (gl) systems allow therapists to conduct virtual exercise supervision sessions, monitor patient adherence through app-based exercise tracking, and deliver follow-up care to individuals who may have difficulty traveling to clinics due to geographic, transportation, or mobility limitations. While virtual care does not replace hands-on treatment when manual interventions are required, hybrid care models combining in-person evaluation with remote follow-up sessions are becoming increasingly common in both outpatient and home-based rehabilitation programs.

Robotic-assisted rehabilitation technology is another developing area. Robotic gait-training systems, motorized resistance therapy devices, and movement-guidance equipment are being used in specialized rehabilitation centers to support neurological (gl) recovery and repetitive movement training. These systems help patients perform high-repetition therapeutic movements that may be difficult to achieve manually, particularly in early-stage neurological rehabilitation where consistency of movement patterns is essential for recovery. Therapists play a central role in programming, supervising, and adjusting these technologies to ensure treatments remain clinically appropriate and patient-centered.

Artificial intelligence (AI) (gl) is also beginning to influence rehabilitation analytics. Predictive modeling systems are being developed to analyze patient progress patterns, identify risk factors for delayed recovery, and assist clinicians in selecting treatment progressions based on large-scale outcome data. While AI does not replace clinical judgment, decision-support systems can help therapists identify treatment options, track recovery benchmarks, and evaluate patient progress against broader population-level trends.

Digital documentation systems continue evolving as well. Electronic health record (gl) platforms increasingly integrate automated outcome-measure tracking, clinical decision prompts, and streamlined documentation templates that reduce administrative workload while improving data consistency. Therapists who develop efficient documentation workflows using these digital systems often spend less time on administrative tasks and more time on direct patient care.

Technology adoption in rehabilitation is not uniform across all practice settings, and the profession continues to emphasize that technological tools are designed to enhance—not replace—the therapeutic relationship between clinician and patient. Successful integration depends on clinicians understanding both the capabilities and limitations of emerging systems while maintaining patient-centered care principles.

Looking forward, rehabilitation technology is expected to expand in several directions: improved wearable movement analytics, expanded remote care platforms, more accessible robotic training tools, and increasingly sophisticated predictive analytics systems. Therapists who remain open to learning new technologies and integrating digital tools into treatment planning will likely find themselves well positioned within evolving healthcare delivery models.

Despite these advancements, the essential foundation of physical therapy remains unchanged. Patients recover through guided movement, therapeutic education, and structured rehabilitation programs designed by skilled clinicians. Technology enhances measurement, access, and efficiency, but the clinical insight, motivation coaching, and individualized care provided by therapists continue to define the profession. Understanding how to combine traditional clinical expertise with emerging technological tools will shape the next generation of rehabilitation practice and open new possibilities for improving patient outcomes across diverse care environments.

Chapter 54

Compensation Modeling Across Practice Settings™

Understanding How Income Structures Differ

Compensation in physical therapy varies significantly depending on clinical setting, geographic region, experience level, and productivity expectations. While salary discussions often focus on national averages, a deeper understanding of how compensation models function across practice environments provides a clearer picture of long-term earning potential and financial planning considerations.

Outpatient Rehabilitation Settings

Outpatient clinics commonly use salary-based compensation models supplemented by productivity incentives. Therapists may receive a base salary with bonus structures tied to visit volume, patient retention rates, or clinic revenue benchmarks. Because outpatient environments often operate on scheduled appointment blocks, income stability is generally predictable, though earnings growth may depend on leadership roles, specialization certifications, or clinic management opportunities.

Hospital-Based Rehabilitation Programs

Hospital rehabilitation roles frequently offer structured salary scales aligned with organizational compensation frameworks. These positions may include comprehensive benefits packages, retirement contributions, and tuition assistance programs that significantly increase total compensation value beyond base salary alone. Hospital settings often emphasize interdisciplinary collaboration and may offer more predictable scheduling compared with some outpatient clinics, though patient acuity levels can vary widely.

Home Health Rehabilitation

Home health compensation often follows per-visit or hybrid salary-plus-visit-pay structures. Therapists may earn higher per-visit rates compared with clinic-based positions, reflecting travel requirements and independent case management responsibilities. Income variability can occur depending on referral volume and geographic travel distances, making scheduling efficiency an important factor in overall earnings stability. Many therapists are drawn to home health roles for the combination of autonomy, flexible scheduling, and strong income potential.

Skilled Nursing and Inpatient Rehabilitation Facilities

Rehabilitation roles in skilled nursing facilities and inpatient rehabilitation hospitals typically offer salary-based compensation with productivity expectations tied to treatment minutes delivered. These settings often provide stable patient volumes, making income predictable, though documentation requirements and regulatory compliance standards can influence daily workflow intensity. Leadership or rehabilitation director roles within these environments often provide additional income growth opportunities.

Specialty and Performance-Based Settings

Therapists working in sports performance centers, specialty rehabilitation programs, or private performance training businesses may encounter compensation structures that combine salary, commission, or independent contractor (gl) income models. These roles sometimes offer higher earning potential tied to program development, athlete training services, or performance consulting, though income stability may vary depending on business volume and market demand.

Long-Term Income Growth Considerations

Income growth within physical therapy careers is influenced not only by experience but also by specialization, leadership responsibilities, geographic mobility, and entrepreneurial initiatives. Therapists who pursue specialty certifications, develop niche clinical expertise, or expand into consulting or ownership roles often create additional earning pathways beyond traditional clinical salaries.

Understanding compensation modeling across practice settings allows clinicians to evaluate career decisions more strategically. Rather than focusing solely on starting salary figures, examining total compensation—including benefits, schedule flexibility, long-term growth potential, and workload expectations—provides a more accurate representation of financial sustainability within the profession.

Chapter 55

Work-Setting Comparison Architecture™

Lifestyle, Income, Stress, and Long-Term Sustainability

Choosing a work setting in physical therapy involves more than selecting a patient population or clinical specialty. Each practice environment carries distinct patterns related to daily workload, scheduling structure, compensation stability, physical demands, and long-term career sustainability. Understanding these structural differences allows therapists to select work environments that align with both professional goals and personal lifestyle priorities.

Outpatient Orthopedic Clinics

Outpatient orthopedic environments often operate on high-volume appointment schedules with consistent patient turnover throughout the day. Therapists frequently treat multiple patients in parallel appointment blocks, requiring strong time-management and documentation efficiency skills. These settings provide excellent exposure to musculoskeletal (gl) conditions, post-surgical rehabilitation, and sports-related injuries, making them attractive for clinicians interested in orthopedic specialization. However, productivity expectations can be higher in some clinics, making workload pacing an important sustainability consideration.

Hospital Acute Care and Inpatient Rehabilitation

Hospital-based rehabilitation roles typically involve treating patients recovering from surgery, trauma, or acute medical conditions. Therapists work as part of interdisciplinary care teams and often see fewer patients per day compared with outpatient environments, though patient acuity levels may be higher. These settings frequently provide stable salaries, strong benefits packages, and structured scheduling systems. The work can be physically demanding but often offers strong team collaboration and varied clinical experiences.

Home Health Physical Therapy

Home health roles provide high levels of scheduling autonomy and independent patient management responsibilities. Therapists travel to patients' homes, evaluate environmental safety conditions, and design treatment plans based on real-world functional mobility (gl) challenges. Compensation per visit is often higher than clinic-based roles, but travel time, scheduling logistics, and geographic coverage areas can influence daily workflow efficiency. Many therapists appreciate the independence and flexible scheduling structure associated with home health practice.

Skilled Nursing Facilities

Skilled nursing environments focus on rehabilitation for older adults recovering from illness, surgery, or functional decline. Therapists frequently treat patients requiring mobility restoration, fall-prevention training, and long-term functional support. These settings often provide stable patient volumes and consistent scheduling, though documentation requirements and regulatory compliance standards can influence administrative workload. Therapists who enjoy working with geriatric populations often find strong alignment within these environments.

Sports Performance and Specialty Clinics

Sports rehabilitation and performance-focused clinics attract therapists interested in athletic injury recovery, return-to-sport programming, and performance optimization. Workflows may include individualized treatment plans, movement analysis, and collaboration with athletic trainers or coaching staff. Income structures may vary depending on clinic ownership models, program development roles, or performance training services offered. These environments often appeal to therapists interested in active, performance-oriented patient populations.

Long-Term Career Sustainability

Work-setting selection is not permanent. Many therapists transition between environments throughout their careers to match evolving professional interests, physical workload preferences, or lifestyle priorities. Early-career clinicians may seek high-exposure learning environments, while mid-career therapists often explore leadership roles or specialty programs, and later-career professionals sometimes transition into consulting, education, or hybrid practice models that reduce full-time patient care intensity.

Understanding how work environments differ in scheduling pace, income structure, physical demands, and long-term sustainability allows therapists to approach career planning strategically. Selecting settings aligned with both professional interests and personal energy patterns often contributes significantly to long-term career satisfaction and professional longevity.

Chapter 56

Pivot Playbook™

Advanced Career Transitions for Physical Therapists

Few healthcare careers remain static over decades, and physical therapy is no exception. As clinicians gain experience, many begin exploring transitions that allow them to apply their expertise in new environments, expand income opportunities, or redesign workload structures to support long-term sustainability. Understanding how career pivots occur within rehabilitation practice allows therapists to make strategic transitions rather than reactive ones.

Clinical Setting Transitions

One of the most common career pivots involves moving between practice settings. Therapists who begin their careers in high-volume outpatient clinics may later transition into hospital-based rehabilitation, home health, specialty neurological rehabilitation programs, or sports performance environments as professional interests evolve. These transitions typically require minimal additional licensure changes, allowing clinicians to adapt their careers without returning to formal degree programs. Exposure to multiple settings over time also broadens clinical skill sets and increases long-term employability.

Specialty Development Pivots

Some therapists pivot by developing specialty expertise in areas such as orthopedic manual therapy, neurological rehabilitation, pediatric therapy, vestibular (gl) rehabilitation, or sports performance training. Specialty certifications and focused continuing education programs often serve as entry points into these transitions. Developing a recognized specialty can open opportunities for leadership roles, advanced clinical positions, consulting work, or teaching responsibilities within educational programs.

Leadership and Administrative Pathways

Career pivots into leadership positions often occur after clinicians develop strong operational understanding of clinical workflow systems, scheduling structures, and interdisciplinary coordination processes. Department director roles, clinical operations management, rehabilitation program leadership, and quality improvement initiatives allow therapists to influence patient care delivery at a systems level rather than solely through individual treatment sessions. These roles often combine clinical insight with operational strategy, offering expanded professional influence.

Entrepreneurial and Ownership Pathways

Some therapists pursue entrepreneurial pivots, establishing private practices, performance training centers, rehabilitation consulting services, or workplace injury-prevention programs. Ownership roles introduce business management responsibilities—staffing, compliance, marketing, and financial planning—but also provide increased autonomy and income potential. Therapists who prepare for entrepreneurship through mentorship, financial education, and operational experience often transition more successfully into ownership roles.

Educational and Consulting Pathways

Experienced clinicians frequently pivot into academic teaching roles, clinical education coordination, continuing education instruction, or rehabilitation consulting services. These pathways allow therapists to apply clinical expertise in ways that influence future clinicians and healthcare systems more broadly. Many professionals combine part-time teaching or consulting work with ongoing clinical practice, creating hybrid career models that evolve over time.

Strategic Timing of Career Pivots

Career transitions are often most successful when planned intentionally rather than triggered solely by burnout or workplace dissatisfaction. Therapists who monitor professional interests, maintain continuing education engagement, and cultivate professional networks often recognize pivot opportunities earlier and transition with greater confidence. Strategic timing also allows clinicians to build financial stability and professional leverage before making significant career changes.

A long-term rehabilitation career rarely consists of a single role repeated for decades. Instead, it unfolds through a series of adaptive transitions that reflect evolving skills, interests, and life priorities. Therapists who view career pivots as normal stages of professional development—rather than disruptions—often discover that each transition expands both career resilience and long-term professional satisfaction.

Chapter 57

What I Wish I Had Known Before Becoming a Physical Therapist™

Realities That Change How You Prepare for the Profession

Every profession looks different from the inside than it does from the outside, and physical therapy is no exception. Many students enter physical therapy programs with strong motivation to help patients regain mobility, recover from injury, and return to meaningful daily activities. Those motivations are well founded. Rehabilitation work is often deeply meaningful, highly visible in its impact, and intellectually engaging. Yet there are operational, financial, and lifestyle realities that many clinicians only fully understand after entering the profession. Knowing these factors earlier can dramatically change how students prepare, how new clinicians approach early career decisions, and how long-term career satisfaction develops.

I Wish I Had Known How Much Documentation Shapes the Day

Students often expect patient care to dominate the entire clinical workday, but documentation requirements (gl) represent a significant portion of professional time. Evaluation reports, treatment notes, progress reports, discharge summaries, and insurance justification documentation all require detailed clinical explanation. Efficient documentation habits become just as important as clinical skill, and clinicians who develop structured note-writing systems early often experience far less after-hours workload pressure. Many therapists eventually realize that documentation efficiency is not a minor administrative skill—it is a core professional competency that directly affects stress levels, productivity expectations, and overall work-life balance.

I Wish I Had Known That Work Setting Matters More Than Job Title

Two therapists with identical degrees and licenses may experience completely different daily careers depending on work setting. Outpatient orthopedic clinics, inpatient rehabilitation hospitals, skilled nursing facilities, home health roles, and sports performance programs operate with distinct scheduling models, productivity expectations, compensation structures, and patient acuity levels. Many clinicians initially evaluate career choices based primarily on the profession itself rather than the environment in which the work is performed. Over time, therapists often discover that long-term satisfaction is influenced as much by workplace structure as by the profession itself.

I Wish I Had Known That Productivity Metrics Influence Workflow More Than I Expected

Healthcare systems operate within reimbursement-driven financial models, and many rehabilitation environments track productivity metrics (gl) such as patient visit volume, billable treatment minutes, or documentation completion timelines. These metrics are not inherently negative—they help organizations maintain operational stability—but they do influence daily workflow pace. Understanding productivity expectations early allows therapists to evaluate whether specific work environments align with their preferred pacing and workload patterns before accepting positions.

I Wish I Had Known That Career Flexibility Is Greater Than It First Appears

Many students assume that choosing physical therapy means committing to a single type of clinical role for decades. In reality, the profession offers extensive flexibility across clinical settings, specialty populations, teaching roles, consulting opportunities, leadership pathways, and entrepreneurial ventures. Therapists frequently move between outpatient care, hospital systems, home health services, performance training, education, or administrative roles as their careers evolve. Recognizing this flexibility earlier helps reduce the pressure of feeling that the first job choice permanently defines the entire career.

I Wish I Had Known How Important Mentorship Would Be

Mentorship relationships often accelerate professional growth far more than clinicians initially expect. Experienced therapists provide practical insights about workflow management, treatment progression decision-making, documentation strategies, and workplace navigation that are difficult to learn from textbooks alone. Clinicians who intentionally seek mentorship early often avoid common early-career mistakes and gain confidence more quickly than those attempting to navigate early practice independently.

I Wish I Had Known That Physical Sustainability Requires Intentional Planning

Physical therapy is an active profession that requires sustained standing, demonstration of exercises, and occasional patient lifting assistance during mobility training. While training programs emphasize body mechanics (gl), many clinicians underestimate how important personal conditioning routines are for long-term career sustainability. Therapists who maintain strength training, mobility routines, and injury-prevention practices often experience fewer musculoskeletal (gl) strain issues over time and maintain higher long-term physical resilience.

I Wish I Had Known That Financial Planning Should Start Before Graduation

Educational investment for physical therapy programs can be significant, and many clinicians wish they had spent more time analyzing loan structures, repayment strategies, and long-term compensation modeling before entering the profession. Early financial awareness does not discourage entry into the field; instead, it allows students to make informed decisions about school selection, geographic employment options, and repayment planning strategies that reduce long-term financial stress.

I Wish I Had Known That Confidence Develops Gradually, Not Immediately

New clinicians sometimes expect to feel fully confident immediately after graduation, yet professional confidence typically develops through repeated patient encounters, mentorship feedback, and clinical experience accumulation over the first several years of practice. Understanding that the early learning curve is normal helps reduce unnecessary self-pressure and allows clinicians to focus on steady skill development rather than unrealistic expectations of immediate mastery.

I Wish I Had Known That Career Satisfaction Depends on Alignment, Not Prestige

The reputation of a profession or specialty does not automatically guarantee personal satisfaction. Therapists who select work environments aligned with their preferred pace, patient population interests, and lifestyle priorities often report higher long-term satisfaction than those who select roles based solely on prestige or perceived expectations. Alignment between daily tasks and personal energy patterns ultimately determines whether careers feel sustainable over time.

I Wish I Had Known That Patient Motivation Is Part of the Job

Clinical training often focuses heavily on anatomy, biomechanics, and treatment techniques, yet a significant portion of rehabilitation success depends on patient motivation and adherence to home exercise programs. Therapists quickly learn that designing the "perfect" treatment plan is only part of the process; helping patients stay engaged, consistent, and confident throughout recovery often determines real-world outcomes. Developing communication strategies that encourage long-term adherence becomes a critical professional skill that many clinicians only fully appreciate after entering practice.

I Wish I Had Known That Communication Skills Influence Outcomes as Much as Clinical Skill

Patients often arrive in therapy with anxiety, frustration, or uncertainty about recovery timelines. The ability to explain treatment goals clearly, set realistic expectations, and maintain supportive therapeutic relationships frequently influences both patient satisfaction and clinical outcomes. Clinicians who invest early in patient education techniques, motivational interviewing (gl) approaches, and clear expectation-setting often find that treatment progress improves when patients understand both the purpose and process of rehabilitation.

I Wish I Had Known That Not Every Day Feels Dramatic — and That's a Good Thing

Many people enter healthcare expecting constant high-intensity clinical moments, but much of rehabilitation involves steady, incremental progress rather than dramatic breakthroughs. Improvement often occurs gradually over weeks or months of consistent effort. Understanding this early helps clinicians develop patience with long-term recovery timelines and recognize the value of cumulative small improvements that ultimately restore patient independence.

I Wish I Had Known That Workplace Culture Strongly Shapes Job Satisfaction

Two positions with similar compensation and patient populations can feel entirely different depending on workplace culture, leadership style, and team collaboration dynamics. Supportive mentorship environments, reasonable scheduling expectations, and strong interdisciplinary collaboration often contribute more to long-term job satisfaction than compensation differences alone. Evaluating organizational culture during interviews becomes an important career decision skill that many clinicians only learn after their first few job experiences.

I Wish I Had Known That Burnout Prevention Starts Early, Not After Exhaustion

Burnout rarely develops overnight; it accumulates gradually when scheduling intensity, documentation pressure, and physical workload consistently exceed recovery time. Therapists who establish sustainable pacing habits early—efficient documentation workflows, physical conditioning routines, and realistic scheduling discussions with supervisors—often maintain higher long-term career satisfaction. Preventive sustainability practices are far easier to establish early than to rebuild after chronic fatigue has developed.

I Wish I Had Known That Networking Is a Career Skill, Not Just a Social Activity

Professional opportunities frequently arise through relationships formed during clinical rotations, professional association involvement, mentorship connections, and continuing education programs. Maintaining professional networks helps clinicians learn about new opportunities, specialty training programs, and leadership roles that may not always be publicly advertised. Early-career therapists who remain engaged with professional communities often discover that career mobility becomes significantly easier over time.

I Wish I Had Known That Continuing Education Shapes Career Direction

Continuing education requirements (gl) are often viewed as licensure obligations, but the courses clinicians select frequently determine long-term specialization pathways. Therapists who intentionally select training aligned with specialty interests gradually build expertise that differentiates them professionally. Over time, these targeted educational choices influence both career opportunities and income potential.

I Wish I Had Known That Career Growth Is Not Always Linear

Many clinicians assume career progression follows a straightforward upward trajectory, yet healthcare careers often involve lateral transitions between work settings, specialty pivots, leadership opportunities, or hybrid roles combining clinical care with education or consulting. Recognizing early that career paths evolve through multiple transitions allows clinicians to remain open to opportunities that may not fit traditional promotion models but still contribute to long-term professional growth.

I Wish I Had Known That Professional Identity Evolves Over Time

The way therapists view their roles changes as experience accumulates. Early-career clinicians often focus on mastering clinical techniques, while mid-career professionals frequently expand into mentorship, leadership, or specialty expertise roles. Later-career therapists often prioritize sustainability, consulting, teaching, or strategic program development.

Understanding that professional identity evolves reduces pressure to "figure everything out" immediately and allows clinicians to grow naturally into different stages of professional contribution.

I Wish I Had Known That Small Systems Create Long-Term Success

Daily habits—organized documentation routines, consistent patient education methods, scheduled recovery time, and ongoing professional learning—may seem minor individually but accumulate into powerful career sustainability systems over time. Therapists who build small, repeatable systems early often find that long-term professional success develops through consistency rather than dramatic career changes.

I Wish I Had Known That Time Management Determines Stress Levels More Than Workload Alone

Many clinicians assume stress is driven primarily by patient volume, yet early in practice it becomes clear that time management systems strongly influence daily pressure levels. Therapists who structure documentation timing, patient preparation routines, and treatment planning workflows efficiently often manage higher caseloads with less stress than clinicians working at similar volumes without structured systems. Learning how to organize clinical workflows early significantly improves long-term workday sustainability.

I Wish I Had Known That Early Job Choices Do Not Permanently Define My Career

Graduating therapists sometimes feel intense pressure to choose the "perfect" first job, fearing that early employment decisions will permanently shape their professional trajectory.

In reality, physical therapy careers are highly mobile across practice settings, specialty areas, and organizational structures. Early roles primarily serve as learning environments, and many clinicians transition between settings within the first several years as their interests and priorities become clearer. Understanding this flexibility reduces unnecessary pressure during the job selection process.

I Wish I Had Known That Clinical Reasoning Develops Through Exposure, Not Just Study

Academic preparation provides strong foundational knowledge, but clinical reasoning skills deepen primarily through repeated patient encounters and reflection on treatment outcomes. Each patient presentation introduces variables that cannot always be fully simulated in classroom settings. Therapists who actively reflect on clinical decisions, seek feedback from experienced colleagues, and analyze treatment outcomes often develop clinical confidence more rapidly than those who rely solely on memorized protocols.

I Wish I Had Known That Financial Growth Often Requires Strategic Movement, Not Waiting

Salary growth in many healthcare systems occurs gradually through standard pay-scale increases. Therapists who periodically evaluate compensation structures across practice settings, pursue specialty certifications, or accept leadership responsibilities often accelerate income growth more effectively than those who rely exclusively on tenure-based raises. Strategic career mobility, when approached thoughtfully, can play a meaningful role in long-term financial planning.

I Wish I Had Known That Interdisciplinary Collaboration Is a Daily Skill

While educational programs emphasize team-based care, many clinicians are surprised by how frequently collaboration with nurses, physicians, occupational therapists, speech-language pathologists, case managers, and social workers occurs in daily practice. Effective communication across disciplines improves discharge planning, treatment coordination, and patient safety. Therapists who develop strong interdisciplinary communication habits early often become key contributors to rehabilitation teams.

I Wish I Had Known That Professional Confidence Is Built Through Consistency, Not Perfection

New clinicians sometimes expect to feel completely confident before making independent treatment decisions, yet confidence typically develops through consistent practice rather than waiting for perfect certainty. Therapists who approach early practice as a learning phase—seeking feedback, refining evaluation approaches, and gradually expanding decision-making independence—often build professional confidence more sustainably than those who delay action until they feel fully certain.

I Wish I Had Known That Mentorship Relationships Can Change Career Trajectories

Mentors often introduce early-career clinicians to specialty areas, leadership opportunities, or professional development pathways they might not have discovered independently. Maintaining relationships with experienced clinicians, former instructors, and clinical supervisors frequently opens doors to career advancement opportunities that may not appear through traditional job-search channels. Mentorship is not only educational—it is also a powerful career navigation tool.

I Wish I Had Known That Patient Outcomes Are Often Nonlinear

Recovery rarely follows perfectly predictable timelines. Some patients progress rapidly, while others require extended rehabilitation periods influenced by medical complexity, social factors, or adherence challenges. Understanding that progress variability is normal helps clinicians maintain realistic expectations and reduces frustration when recovery timelines differ from initial projections.

I Wish I Had Known That Long-Term Career Satisfaction Requires Periodic Reassessment

Professional interests, lifestyle priorities, and physical workload preferences change over time. Therapists who periodically reassess their work settings, specialty interests, and scheduling preferences often maintain higher long-term satisfaction than those who remain in roles that no longer align with evolving priorities. Career reassessment is not a sign of instability—it is a normal component of long-term professional growth.

I Wish I Had Known That Small Adjustments Early Prevent Large Problems Later

Minor habits—consistent documentation timing, proactive communication with supervisors, maintaining personal physical conditioning, and continuing education engagement—may appear insignificant in the short term but accumulate into powerful long-term career sustainability factors.

Clinicians who implement these small adjustments early often avoid larger stressors later in their careers.

I Wish I Had Known That Early Career Pace Feels Faster Than School Preparation Suggests

Academic programs prepare students thoroughly for clinical decision-making, yet the pace of full-time clinical practice often feels faster than many new graduates initially expect. Multiple patients scheduled back-to-back, real-time documentation responsibilities, interdisciplinary communication, and scheduling adjustments require rapid workflow adaptation. Therapists who anticipate this transition period and allow themselves time to develop pacing systems typically adapt more comfortably during the first year of practice.

I Wish I Had Known That Asking for Help Is a Professional Strength

New clinicians sometimes hesitate to ask experienced colleagues for input because they want to appear independent. In practice, seeking guidance when encountering unfamiliar cases improves both patient care and professional development. Healthcare environments function best when clinicians collaborate openly, and therapists who ask thoughtful questions early often accelerate their learning curves significantly.

I Wish I Had Known That Reputation Builds Quietly but Powerfully

Professional reputation develops through reliability, communication quality, teamwork, and consistency rather than through single standout moments. Therapists who consistently complete documentation on time, communicate clearly with team members, and provide dependable patient care gradually build reputations that influence promotion opportunities, leadership invitations, and referral relationships. Many career opportunities arise because colleagues trust a clinician's reliability over time.

I Wish I Had Known That Career Satisfaction Is Strongly Influenced by Scheduling Structure

Beyond compensation and patient population, scheduling design plays a major role in daily job satisfaction. Appointment spacing, documentation time allocation, commute patterns, and workload predictability all influence long-term sustainability. Therapists who evaluate scheduling structures carefully during job selection often find greater long-term alignment than those focusing solely on salary figures.

I Wish I Had Known That Emotional Energy Is Part of the Workload

Physical therapy involves working closely with individuals experiencing pain, injury recovery, or functional limitations, and emotional engagement with patients can be both rewarding and demanding. Supporting patients through frustration, setbacks, or slow progress requires emotional presence in addition to clinical expertise. Clinicians who develop recovery routines outside work—exercise, hobbies, social connection, or relaxation practices—often maintain stronger long-term resilience.

I Wish I Had Known That Leadership Opportunities Begin Earlier Than Expected

Leadership in healthcare is not limited to formal management titles. Early-career therapists often have opportunities to lead quality improvement initiatives, assist with onboarding new staff, contribute to workflow optimization projects, or mentor students during clinical rotations. Engaging in these opportunities early helps clinicians develop leadership skills that support future advancement.

I Wish I Had Known That Technology Will Continue Changing Practice

Digital documentation systems, wearable rehabilitation monitoring tools, tele-rehabilitation platforms, and data analytics systems are increasingly influencing rehabilitation practice. Therapists who remain adaptable to technological change often find that learning new systems becomes easier when approached with curiosity rather than resistance. Technology adoption typically enhances efficiency and measurement accuracy when integrated thoughtfully into clinical workflows.

I Wish I Had Known That Long-Term Career Growth Depends on Strategic Learning Choices

Continuing education requirements ensure ongoing licensure, but selecting courses intentionally—aligned with specialty interests or emerging healthcare needs—gradually shapes long-term career positioning. Therapists who approach continuing education strategically often build expertise that expands both career mobility and income potential.

I Wish I Had Known That Career Longevity Is Built Through Balance, Not Endurance Alone

Some clinicians initially believe that professional success comes from working at maximum capacity indefinitely. Over time, many discover that long-term career sustainability depends on balancing productivity, recovery, physical conditioning, and professional development. Therapists who maintain sustainable pacing habits often enjoy longer, more satisfying careers than those who attempt to operate continuously at peak intensity.

I Wish I Had Known That Alignment Matters More Than Expectations

External expectations—from peers, mentors, or perceived prestige—can sometimes influence career decisions more than personal alignment. Therapists who periodically reassess whether their current roles match their interests, preferred work environments, and lifestyle priorities often maintain stronger long-term satisfaction. Alignment between daily responsibilities and personal strengths ultimately determines whether careers remain energizing or gradually become draining.

I Wish I Had Known That Early Career Comparisons Can Be Misleading

New clinicians often compare their speed, confidence, or treatment creativity to therapists who have practiced for ten or twenty years. These comparisons can create unnecessary self-doubt during the early learning phase. Experienced clinicians operate from thousands of patient encounters and refined pattern recognition (gl) developed over time. Understanding that early-career growth naturally involves a steep learning curve helps clinicians focus on steady improvement rather than unrealistic comparisons.

I Wish I Had Known That Communication With Referring Providers Matters More Than I Expected

Therapists frequently interact with referring physicians, surgeons, nurse practitioners, and other healthcare providers to update treatment progress and adjust care plans. Clear, concise communication strengthens referral relationships and helps ensure continuity of care across disciplines. Clinicians who develop strong professional communication habits early often build referral trust that influences long-term patient volume and professional reputation.

I Wish I Had Known That Not All Stress Comes From Patient Care

Administrative responsibilities, scheduling variability, productivity expectations, and insurance authorization processes often contribute to professional stress as much as clinical workload. Recognizing these operational factors early allows therapists to develop workflow systems that reduce administrative pressure and maintain focus on patient care priorities.

I Wish I Had Known That Professional Boundaries Protect Long-Term Sustainability

Healthcare professionals often feel a strong desire to help every patient as much as possible, sometimes extending work hours or taking on excessive caseloads. While dedication is admirable, sustainable careers require maintaining professional boundaries that protect personal time, physical recovery, and long-term health. Therapists who learn to balance commitment with realistic workload limits often maintain stronger career longevity.

I Wish I Had Known That Career Mobility Is a Strength of the Profession

Physical therapy licensure allows movement across many clinical settings with minimal retraining compared with some healthcare professions. This mobility enables therapists to adjust roles when interests change, family needs shift, or lifestyle priorities evolve. Recognizing this flexibility early helps clinicians view career decisions as adjustable rather than permanent.

I Wish I Had Known That Mentoring Others Reinforces My Own Learning

When therapists begin mentoring students or new clinicians, they often discover that teaching reinforces their own clinical reasoning skills. Explaining treatment rationale, demonstrating evaluation techniques, and answering questions deepens understanding and strengthens professional confidence. Teaching is not only a way to give back; it also strengthens personal expertise.

I Wish I Had Known That Long-Term Financial Planning Requires Active Attention

Healthcare careers provide stable income potential, but long-term financial growth depends on active planning—loan repayment strategies, retirement contributions, and career positioning decisions that influence compensation growth. Therapists who begin financial planning early often gain greater long-term flexibility in career decision-making.

I Wish I Had Known That Job Satisfaction Often Depends on Leadership Quality

Supportive leadership environments that provide mentorship, reasonable scheduling expectations, and clear communication frequently contribute more to job satisfaction than small salary differences. Evaluating leadership style during interviews—through questions about mentorship structure, productivity expectations, and team culture—helps clinicians make more informed employment decisions.

I Wish I Had Known That Career Direction Clarifies Through Experience

Many clinicians expect to know their long-term specialty interests immediately after graduation, yet preferences often emerge only after exposure to diverse patient populations and work settings. Allowing time for exploration during the early years of practice helps therapists discover areas of genuine professional interest before committing to specialization pathways.

I Wish I Had Known That Sustainable Careers Are Built Intentionally

Long-term career satisfaction rarely occurs by accident. Therapists who periodically reassess professional goals, continue developing skills, maintain professional networks, and adjust work environments when necessary often create careers that remain both meaningful and sustainable over decades. Intentional career design, rather than passive progression, becomes one of the most valuable professional habits clinicians can develop.

I Wish I Had Known That Confidence and Competence Grow at Different Speeds

In the early months of practice, many therapists discover that competence often develops before confidence catches up. Clinicians may already be making sound clinical decisions while still feeling uncertain internally. Recognizing this gap is important, because it prevents new therapists from misinterpreting normal early-career uncertainty as lack of ability. Confidence tends to rise gradually as repeated patient encounters confirm that evaluation processes, treatment progressions, and patient communication strategies are working effectively.

I Wish I Had Known That Career Direction Is Influenced by Exposure

The clinical populations therapists encounter early in their careers often shape long-term specialty interests. A clinician exposed primarily to orthopedic rehabilitation may initially assume that orthopedics will define their career, only to later discover interest in neurological rehabilitation, pediatrics, or sports performance when given broader exposure. Seeking diverse early-career experiences allows therapists to make specialty decisions based on informed preference rather than limited initial exposure.

I Wish I Had Known That Professional Growth Requires Saying Yes to Learning Opportunities

Invitations to assist with program development, participate in clinical committees, mentor students, or attend specialty training workshops sometimes appear unexpectedly. Early-career therapists who accept these learning opportunities often gain experience that accelerates leadership readiness and professional positioning. Growth frequently occurs when clinicians step slightly outside their comfort zones to explore new responsibilities.

I Wish I Had Known That Small Professional Habits Shape Long-Term Reputation

Consistent punctuality, timely documentation, organized communication, and respectful collaboration with colleagues may appear routine, but these habits form the foundation of professional reputation over time. Supervisors, peers, and referral providers often remember reliability long after individual clinical encounters fade from memory. Many career advancement opportunities arise because colleagues trust a clinician's consistency.

I Wish I Had Known That Career Satisfaction Is Strongly Influenced by Patient Population Fit

Some therapists thrive working with athletes returning to sport, others prefer geriatric mobility rehabilitation, neurological recovery, pediatric development, or chronic pain management programs. Discovering which patient populations align best with personal communication style, energy patterns, and clinical interests significantly influences long-term career enjoyment. Therapists who identify this alignment early often make more satisfying work-setting decisions.

I Wish I Had Known That Professional Resilience Comes From Recovery Habits Outside Work

Healthcare professionals often focus heavily on patient recovery while overlooking their own recovery needs. Regular exercise, sufficient sleep, personal hobbies, and time away from clinical environments help maintain physical and emotional resilience. Therapists who build consistent recovery routines often sustain higher long-term energy levels and professional engagement.

I Wish I Had Known That Learning Never Truly Slows Down

Healthcare knowledge evolves continuously, and rehabilitation techniques, treatment technologies, and care delivery models change over time. Therapists who remain curious, attend continuing education programs, and engage with professional communities often find that the profession remains intellectually stimulating throughout their careers. Lifelong learning is not only a requirement for licensure; it is a source of ongoing professional satisfaction.

I Wish I Had Known That Leadership Is Often Informal Before It Becomes Formal

Many therapists begin demonstrating leadership through mentoring students, assisting colleagues with clinical challenges, or helping improve workflow systems before ever holding official leadership titles. Recognizing these informal leadership opportunities allows clinicians to develop management and communication skills early, positioning them for future formal leadership roles if desired.

I Wish I Had Known That Career Longevity Is Built Through Strategic Adjustments

Over decades of practice, therapists often adjust work settings, scheduling intensity, specialty focus, or professional responsibilities to maintain sustainability. Viewing career changes as strategic adjustments rather than disruptions helps clinicians remain flexible as life circumstances and professional interests evolve.

I Wish I Had Known That Alignment Is the Most Reliable Predictor of Long-Term Satisfaction

Ultimately, the therapists who report the highest long-term satisfaction are not always those with the highest salaries or most prestigious job titles. They are often those whose daily responsibilities align closely with their strengths, interests, and preferred work environments. Understanding personal alignment early allows clinicians to design careers that remain both meaningful and sustainable over time.

I Wish I Had Known That The First Year Feels Like Learning a Second Language

Entering full-time clinical practice often feels similar to learning a new professional language. Therapists must integrate clinical terminology, documentation systems, insurance authorization requirements, scheduling software, interdisciplinary communication protocols, and treatment planning processes simultaneously. Even highly prepared graduates frequently need several months before these operational systems begin to feel routine. Understanding that this adjustment period is normal helps new clinicians remain patient with themselves during the early transition from school to practice.

I Wish I Had Known That Feedback Accelerates Growth

Constructive feedback from experienced clinicians, supervisors, and colleagues often shortens the learning curve dramatically. Therapists who actively request feedback on evaluation techniques, treatment progression decisions, and patient communication approaches often develop clinical confidence more quickly than those who rely solely on self-assessment. Feedback is not a critique of competence; it is one of the most effective professional growth tools available.

I Wish I Had Known That Career Satisfaction Is Closely Linked to Team Dynamics

Working within supportive teams where communication is open, mentorship is accessible, and workloads are shared effectively often contributes more to job satisfaction than any single job benefit. Therapists who evaluate team culture during interviews—asking about mentorship programs, collaborative rounds, and communication expectations—often gain clearer insight into the daily experience of the role.

I Wish I Had Known That Some Skills Become Easier Faster Than Expected

Certain professional tasks that initially feel difficult—such as patient education explanations, documentation phrasing, or treatment session pacing—often become routine surprisingly quickly with repetition. Recognizing that early discomfort is temporary helps clinicians maintain confidence while mastering new responsibilities.

I Wish I Had Known That Career Opportunities Often Appear Through Relationships

Many job openings, leadership invitations, and consulting opportunities arise through professional relationships rather than public job postings. Therapists who maintain connections with former classmates, clinical instructors, continuing education colleagues, and professional association members often hear about opportunities earlier than those working in isolation. Networking is less about self-promotion and more about staying connected to professional communities.

I Wish I Had Known That Professional Growth Includes Learning When to Slow Down

Ambitious clinicians sometimes attempt to accept every opportunity simultaneously—high patient volumes, additional committees, extra training programs, and extended work hours. Over time, many discover that sustainable growth involves choosing learning opportunities strategically rather than attempting to pursue everything at once. Focused development often produces stronger expertise than overextended participation.

I Wish I Had Known That Early Career Stress Often Decreases Faster Than Expected

The first several months of practice can feel intense as clinicians adapt to workflow pace and decision-making responsibility. However, as documentation routines stabilize, patient education explanations become familiar, and treatment planning becomes more intuitive, stress levels often decrease significantly. Understanding that the early adjustment period is temporary helps new clinicians remain patient with the learning process.

I Wish I Had Known That Personal Health Habits Influence Professional Endurance

Because the profession involves physical activity throughout the day, maintaining personal strength, flexibility, and recovery routines significantly affects long-term sustainability. Therapists who treat their own conditioning as seriously as their patients' often experience fewer cumulative strain injuries and maintain higher long-term physical energy.

I Wish I Had Known That Career Direction Clarifies Through Action

Some clinicians delay pursuing specialty certifications, leadership opportunities, or advanced training because they feel uncertain about long-term direction. In reality, taking exploratory steps—attending workshops, participating in specialty clinics, or assisting in program development—often clarifies career interests more effectively than prolonged indecision. Action frequently produces clarity.

I Wish I Had Known That Long-Term Fulfillment Comes From Growth, Not Stability Alone

While job stability is valuable, many therapists discover that ongoing learning, evolving responsibilities, and periodic career adjustments contribute more to long-term fulfillment than remaining in unchanged roles. Careers that include growth, new challenges, and expanding expertise often remain energizing across decades of practice.

I Wish I Had Known That Early Career Discomfort Often Signals Growth

During the first years of practice, therapists frequently encounter situations that feel unfamiliar—complex patient presentations, fast-paced scheduling days, or treatment planning challenges that require deeper clinical reasoning. While these moments can initially feel uncomfortable, they often represent the environments where the most rapid professional growth occurs. Recognizing discomfort as part of the development process helps clinicians remain engaged rather than discouraged during challenging periods.

I Wish I Had Known That Communication Style Evolves With Experience

New clinicians often focus intensely on explaining every technical detail of treatment plans. Over time, therapists learn how to tailor communication to each patient's needs, simplifying explanations while maintaining clarity and confidence. Developing flexible communication styles improves patient engagement, strengthens therapeutic relationships, and enhances treatment adherence across diverse patient populations.

I Wish I Had Known That Career Fulfillment Often Comes From Small Patient Wins

Major recovery milestones—returning to work after injury or regaining independent mobility—are deeply rewarding, but many therapists discover that daily professional satisfaction often comes from smaller progress moments: a patient achieving a new range-of-motion goal, walking slightly farther than the previous session, or regaining confidence in everyday movement tasks. Appreciating these incremental successes helps maintain motivation throughout long rehabilitation timelines.

I Wish I Had Known That Long-Term Career Satisfaction Requires Periodic Adjustment

Therapists who remain open to adjusting work settings, scheduling intensity, or specialty focus often maintain higher long-term engagement than those who attempt to remain in the same role indefinitely. Career adjustment does not represent instability; it reflects responsiveness to changing professional interests, physical workload preferences, and evolving life priorities.

I Wish I Had Known That Building Professional Confidence Takes Time

Confidence is not a single milestone achieved after licensure. It develops gradually as therapists observe patient progress, refine evaluation strategies, and gain repeated exposure to diverse clinical scenarios. Recognizing that confidence builds over years rather than months helps clinicians remain patient with their own professional development.

I Wish I Had Known That Patient Relationships Are Central to the Profession

Rehabilitation often involves working with patients over multiple weeks or months, creating ongoing therapeutic relationships that differ from short-term clinical encounters in some healthcare roles. These longer relationships allow therapists to witness meaningful functional recovery, but they also require consistent empathy, communication, and emotional presence. Understanding this relational aspect of the profession helps clinicians prepare for both its rewards and responsibilities.

I Wish I Had Known That Early Career Learning Is Exponential

The first few years of practice often involve rapid skill acquisition as therapists encounter diverse patient cases and treatment scenarios. Learning that feels slow during individual days often accumulates quickly across months of practice. Many clinicians are surprised by how much their clinical reasoning and workflow efficiency improve within the first several years when they actively engage in learning opportunities.

I Wish I Had Known That Professional Identity Develops Gradually

New clinicians sometimes expect to feel fully "established" in their professional identities immediately after graduation. In reality, professional identity evolves through clinical experience, mentorship relationships, and exposure to different patient populations. Over time, therapists naturally refine their professional interests, treatment philosophies, and career direction.

I Wish I Had Known That Sustainable Careers Depend on Recovery as Much as Effort

Healthcare professionals often focus heavily on effort—seeing more patients, learning more techniques, working longer hours—but long-term success also depends on recovery. Adequate rest, physical conditioning, and personal time outside clinical work help maintain the energy required for decades of patient care. Therapists who prioritize recovery habits early often sustain higher long-term career endurance.

I Wish I Had Known That Choosing the Right Environment Matters as Much as Choosing the Right Profession

The physical therapy profession offers many rewarding opportunities, but job satisfaction often depends heavily on workplace structure, team culture, scheduling expectations, and leadership style. Therapists who evaluate employment environments carefully—looking beyond job titles alone—often find positions that align more closely with their long-term professional goals and lifestyle preferences.

I Wish I Had Known That Clinical Confidence Comes From Repetition, Not Perfection

Early in practice, many therapists believe they must deliver flawless treatment sessions to feel competent. Over time, clinicians discover that professional confidence grows primarily through repetition—evaluating many patients, refining treatment approaches, and observing recovery patterns across diverse cases. Each patient encounter adds to a growing internal database of experience that strengthens decision-making confidence far more effectively than waiting to feel "fully ready."

I Wish I Had Known That Learning to Pace the Workday Is a Professional Skill

Managing energy throughout a full clinical schedule requires intentional pacing. Therapists who learn how to balance physically demanding sessions with lighter treatment blocks, maintain hydration, and organize documentation timing strategically often finish workdays with significantly less fatigue. Energy management becomes an essential skill for sustaining long-term productivity and physical endurance.

I Wish I Had Known That Career Direction Becomes Clearer Through Exposure to Different Settings

Experiencing multiple clinical environments—outpatient clinics, hospital rehabilitation programs, home health roles, or specialty rehabilitation centers—often clarifies long-term career preferences. Exposure allows therapists to understand how workflow structures, patient populations, and scheduling patterns differ across settings. Many clinicians discover their strongest professional alignment only after working in more than one environment.

I Wish I Had Known That Professional Growth Includes Learning Operational Systems

Understanding scheduling workflows, documentation systems, reimbursement structures, and referral processes contributes significantly to career advancement. Therapists who understand how healthcare systems function often position themselves for leadership roles, program development opportunities, or entrepreneurial ventures more effectively than those focusing solely on clinical technique development.

I Wish I Had Known That Patient Education Is a Core Treatment Tool

While exercise prescription and manual therapy techniques receive significant attention during training, patient education often plays an equally powerful role in treatment success. Helping patients understand injury mechanisms, recovery timelines, and self-management strategies improves adherence and long-term outcomes. Therapists who develop strong educational communication habits often see more consistent patient progress.

I Wish I Had Known That Career Opportunities Often Expand Unexpectedly

Many therapists begin their careers focused solely on patient care, only to later discover opportunities in leadership, teaching, consulting, research collaboration, or specialty program development. Remaining open to unexpected opportunities allows clinicians to explore professional pathways they may not have initially considered but later find highly fulfilling.

I Wish I Had Known That Mentorship Relationships Continue Throughout the Career

Mentorship does not end after the first job. Even experienced clinicians benefit from consulting peers with different specialties, learning from senior leaders, or collaborating with interdisciplinary professionals. Ongoing mentorship relationships continue to support professional growth long after early-career stages.

I Wish I Had Known That Professional Reputation Compounds Over Time

Small professional habits—meeting deadlines, communicating clearly, supporting colleagues, and maintaining ethical standards—accumulate into long-term professional reputation. As reputations strengthen, therapists often find that referral opportunities, leadership invitations, and consulting roles emerge more frequently.

I Wish I Had Known That Long-Term Career Satisfaction Is Built Through Intentional Design

Careers that remain satisfying over decades are rarely accidental. Therapists who periodically evaluate whether their roles align with evolving interests, physical workload preferences, and lifestyle priorities often make strategic adjustments that maintain engagement. Career design is an ongoing process rather than a one-time decision.

I Wish I Had Known That Alignment Ultimately Determines Longevity

At its core, long-term success in physical therapy depends on whether the daily responsibilities of the profession align with personal strengths, interests, and preferred work environments. When alignment exists, clinicians often remain energized by the work even during demanding periods. When alignment is absent, even technically successful careers can feel draining over time. Recognizing the importance of alignment early allows therapists to make career decisions that support both professional success and long-term personal sustainability.

I Wish I Had Known That Early Career Uncertainty Is Normal

Many new clinicians expect to feel completely certain about treatment decisions immediately after graduation. In reality, uncertainty during the early months of practice is a normal part of professional development. Therapists gradually become more comfortable making clinical decisions as they gain experience evaluating diverse patient cases and observing how treatment strategies influence outcomes over time. Recognizing that uncertainty is part of the learning process helps clinicians remain patient with their own development.

I Wish I Had Known That Patient Outcomes Often Require Patience

Some patients progress quickly, while others require extended rehabilitation timelines due to injury severity, underlying medical conditions, or lifestyle factors. Therapists who understand early that recovery is often nonlinear are better prepared to guide patients through setbacks without losing confidence in the rehabilitation process. Patience becomes an essential professional trait that supports both clinician resilience and patient encouragement.

I Wish I Had Known That Workplace Fit Influences Daily Experience More Than Expected

Two therapists performing similar clinical duties can experience vastly different workdays depending on team culture, scheduling expectations, leadership communication, and available mentorship support. Therapists who evaluate workplace fit carefully—asking about mentorship structure, workload expectations, and documentation support systems—often find roles that align more closely with their preferred professional environments.

I Wish I Had Known That Career Development Is Continuous, Not Front-Loaded

Professional learning does not end after licensure or the first few years of practice. Rehabilitation techniques evolve, patient populations change, and healthcare delivery models shift over time. Therapists who approach their careers as ongoing learning journeys often remain more adaptable and engaged than those who expect professional growth to stabilize after early training.

I Wish I Had Known That Professional Confidence Comes From Reflection

Reflecting on patient outcomes, reviewing treatment decisions, and discussing challenging cases with colleagues helps clinicians refine their clinical reasoning skills. Therapists who build reflection habits into their practice often develop stronger decision-making confidence and more efficient treatment planning approaches over time.

I Wish I Had Known That Professional Fulfillment Often Comes From Patient Impact

While compensation, scheduling, and career advancement opportunities matter, many therapists ultimately find that long-term fulfillment comes from witnessing meaningful patient progress—seeing individuals regain independence, return to work, or resume activities they value. These outcomes often become the moments that sustain motivation during demanding periods of practice.

I Wish I Had Known That Career Longevity Requires Flexibility

Healthcare systems, reimbursement models, and workforce demands evolve continuously. Therapists who remain flexible —willing to adjust work settings, develop new specialty skills, or explore leadership opportunities—often maintain greater career resilience than those who resist change. Flexibility becomes a strategic advantage over long professional timelines.

I Wish I Had Known That Strong Professional Relationships Shape Career Opportunities

Supportive colleagues, mentors, supervisors, and professional peers often play key roles in career advancement by sharing knowledge, recommending opportunities, and providing guidance during transitions. Investing in professional relationships early frequently creates networks that support long-term career mobility.

I Wish I Had Known That Long-Term Career Satisfaction Is Built Incrementally

Satisfying careers are rarely created through single large decisions; they develop through many small choices—selecting learning opportunities, building mentorship relationships, adjusting work environments, and maintaining professional curiosity. Over time, these incremental decisions shape careers that remain both meaningful and sustainable.

I Wish I Had Known That Understanding the Profession Deeply Changes How You Enter It

Students who understand the operational, financial, physical, and emotional realities of rehabilitation practice before entering the field often transition more smoothly into professional roles. Awareness allows clinicians to prepare intentionally—developing documentation skills, financial plans, physical conditioning routines, and mentorship connections that support early career success.

I Wish I Had Known That Career Satisfaction Often Depends on How You Structure Your Role

Two therapists working within the same organization can experience very different levels of satisfaction depending on how they structure their responsibilities. Some clinicians negotiate schedules that allow focused patient care blocks followed by dedicated documentation time, while others accept scheduling patterns that create constant time pressure. Learning early that role structure can often be adjusted—through communication with supervisors or thoughtful job selection—helps clinicians shape positions that better match their working style.

I Wish I Had Known That The Profession Rewards Adaptability

Healthcare environments evolve constantly due to regulatory updates, reimbursement model changes, new technology systems, and shifting patient population needs. Therapists who approach change with adaptability rather than resistance often find transitions easier and discover new opportunities that accompany evolving healthcare delivery systems. Adaptability becomes one of the most valuable long-term professional traits.

I Wish I Had Known That Confidence With Patients Develops Faster Than Expected

While clinical decision-making confidence takes time, comfort interacting with patients often develops quickly once therapists begin practicing regularly. Repeating patient education explanations, treatment demonstrations, and motivational coaching conversations builds communication ease that becomes second nature within the first year of practice.

I Wish I Had Known That Professional Growth Is Influenced by the Questions You Ask

Therapists who ask thoughtful questions—about treatment outcomes, workflow efficiency, leadership opportunities, and specialty pathways—often uncover learning opportunities that remain invisible to those who remain passive. Curiosity consistently opens doors to professional development experiences that shape long-term career direction.

I Wish I Had Known That Career Flexibility Protects Long-Term Motivation

Knowing that the profession allows movement between clinical settings, specialty areas, leadership roles, teaching positions, or consulting opportunities reduces the feeling of being locked into a single career structure. Therapists who periodically explore new responsibilities often maintain stronger professional engagement than those who remain in unchanged roles for extended periods.

I Wish I Had Known That Many Career Opportunities Appear Gradually, Not Suddenly

Opportunities such as mentoring roles, leadership positions, specialty program development, or consulting invitations often emerge slowly as clinicians build experience and professional relationships. Recognizing that career growth unfolds over time helps therapists remain patient with their professional development rather than expecting immediate advancement.

I Wish I Had Known That Professional Satisfaction Often Comes From Mastery

As therapists refine their clinical reasoning, develop treatment efficiency, and build strong patient outcomes, daily work often becomes more rewarding. Mastery transforms tasks that once required intense concentration into fluid professional routines, allowing clinicians to focus more fully on patient interaction and treatment creativity.

I Wish I Had Known That Early Career Decisions Benefit From Long-Term Thinking

Considering how early job experiences contribute to long-term skill development, professional networks, and specialty exploration often leads to better career decisions than focusing solely on short-term compensation differences. Positions that provide strong mentorship and learning exposure frequently create greater long-term advantages than slightly higher starting salaries without developmental support.

I Wish I Had Known That The Profession Continues to Offer New Directions

Many clinicians discover career pathways years after graduation that they did not initially know existed—specialty consulting roles, advanced rehabilitation technology integration, academic teaching opportunities, or healthcare operations leadership. Remaining open to emerging directions helps therapists build careers that continue evolving rather than feeling repetitive.

I Wish I Had Known That Alignment Makes the Hard Days Sustainable

Every healthcare career includes demanding days, yet clinicians who feel aligned with their work—valuing patient recovery, movement science, and rehabilitation progress—often find that purpose offsets many of the daily challenges. Alignment between professional responsibilities and personal motivation ultimately determines whether careers remain energizing across decades of practice.

Chapter 58

Glossary

Activities of Daily Living

Activities of Daily Living — Routine self-care tasks such as bathing, dressing, eating, and mobility that are commonly evaluated in rehabilitation planning.

Ambulation

Ambulation — The ability to walk independently or with assistance, frequently assessed during rehabilitation.

Anatomy

Anatomy — The study of the structure of the human body, including muscles, bones, nerves, and organs.

Biomechanics

Biomechanics — The study of how mechanical principles apply to human movement and physical function.

Clinical Reasoning

Clinical Reasoning — The decision-making process clinicians use to evaluate patient conditions and determine treatment strategies.

Compliance

Compliance — The degree to which a patient follows prescribed therapy or treatment recommendations.

Continuing Education Requirements

Continuing Education Requirements — Mandatory educational activities clinicians must complete to maintain professional licensure.

Documentation Systems

Documentation Systems — Electronic or paper systems used to record patient evaluations, treatments, and progress.

Electronic Health Record

Electronic Health Record — A digital version of a patient's medical history maintained by healthcare providers.

Ergonomics

Ergonomics — The science of designing work and activity environments to reduce physical strain and injury risk.

Functional Capacity

Functional Capacity — The level of physical ability an individual can safely perform in daily or occupational tasks.

Geriatric

Geriatric — Relating to healthcare services focused on older adult populations.

Interdisciplinary

Interdisciplinary — Collaboration among professionals from different healthcare specialties working together to manage patient care.

Licensure

Licensure — Official authorization granted by a regulatory body allowing a clinician to practice professionally.

Neurological

Neurological — Relating to the nervous system, including the brain, spinal cord, and nerves.

Pathology

Pathology — The study of diseases and the effects they have on the body.

Physiology

Physiology — The study of how the human body functions at cellular, tissue, and system levels.

Productivity Expectations

Productivity Expectations — Workplace benchmarks that determine how many patients or treatment units a clinician is expected to complete within a specific timeframe.

Regulatory Compliance

Regulatory Compliance — Adherence to laws, regulations, and professional standards governing healthcare practice.

Reimbursement Structures

Reimbursement Structures — Payment systems through which healthcare providers are compensated by insurers or payers for services delivered.

Spinal Cord Injury

Spinal Cord Injury — Damage to the spinal cord that may result in loss of movement, sensation, or function below the injury site.

Specialty Certifications

Specialty Certifications — Advanced credentials demonstrating specialized clinical expertise within a focused area of practice.

Tele-Rehabilitation

Tele-Rehabilitation — Delivery of rehabilitation services through virtual or remote communication technologies.

Traumatic Brain Injury

Traumatic Brain Injury — Brain dysfunction caused by external force, often requiring specialized rehabilitation treatment.

Workload Distribution

Workload Distribution — The allocation of patient caseload responsibilities among clinicians within an organization.

Introduction: 100 Bonus Terms Future Physical Therapists Should Know

Physical therapy is a profession built on movement science, clinical reasoning, documentation precision, and interdisciplinary collaboration. Long before entering graduate training, students who begin learning the language of rehabilitation gain a meaningful advantage: lectures become easier to follow, clinical observations make more sense, and early professional conversations feel less intimidating. Vocabulary familiarity does not make someone a clinician, but it dramatically shortens the learning curve once formal education begins.

The following **100 bonus terms** introduce foundational concepts commonly encountered in physical therapy coursework, clinical rotations, documentation systems, and early professional practice. You are not expected to memorize every definition immediately. Instead, treat this list as a working reference that you revisit periodically as your understanding deepens. Over time, repeated exposure will transform unfamiliar terminology into practical working knowledge that supports both academic success and long-term professional confidence.

100 Bonus Terms for Future Physical Therapists

1. Acute Care — Short-term treatment for severe injuries or illnesses, typically delivered in hospital settings.

2. Adaptive Equipment — Devices designed to help patients perform daily activities more independently.

3. Alignment — Proper positioning of body structures to optimize movement efficiency.

4. Assistive Technology — Tools or systems that improve functional independence for individuals with disabilities.

5. Atrophy — Decrease in muscle size due to inactivity or neurological impairment.

6. Balance Training — Therapeutic exercises aimed at improving stability and fall prevention.

7. Baseline Measurement — Initial assessment values used to track patient progress over time.

8. Body Mechanics — Proper posture and movement strategies used to prevent injury.

9. Care Plan — Structured outline of treatment goals, interventions, and expected outcomes.

10. Case Management — Coordination of healthcare services across providers and settings.

11. Chronic Condition — Long-term health condition requiring ongoing management.

12. Clinical Outcome Measures — Standardized tools used to evaluate treatment effectiveness.

13. Co-Treatment — Collaborative therapy provided by two clinicians simultaneously.

14. Cognitive Impairment — Reduced mental processing affecting memory, reasoning, or attention.

15. Compensatory Strategy — Alternative movement method used to achieve a task when normal function is limited.

16. Contracture — Permanent shortening of muscles or joints that limits movement.

17. Core Stability — Strength and control of trunk muscles that support posture and movement.

18. Degenerative Disease — Condition involving gradual deterioration of body structures.

19. Differential Diagnosis — Process of distinguishing between conditions with similar symptoms.

20. Discharge Planning — Preparation for patient transition from therapy to independent care.

21. Edema — Swelling caused by fluid accumulation in tissues.

22. Endurance Training — Exercises designed to improve cardiovascular stamina.

23. Evidence-Based Practice — Clinical decision-making guided by research, experience, and patient values.

24. Flexibility Training — Exercises designed to increase joint range of motion.

25. Functional Assessment — Evaluation of a patient's ability to perform daily activities.

26. Functional Mobility — Ability to move safely within home or community environments.

27. Gait Analysis — Systematic study of walking patterns.

28. Gross Motor Skills — Large body movements involving major muscle groups.

29. Hand Therapy — Rehabilitation focused on hand and upper-extremity function.

30. Home Exercise Program — Customized exercise plan prescribed for patients to complete outside therapy sessions.

31. Hydration Status — Level of body fluid balance affecting performance and recovery.

32. Immobilization — Restricting movement to allow healing.

33. Impairment — Loss or abnormality of physiological function.

34. Inflammation — Biological response to injury causing redness, swelling, and pain.

35. Joint Stability — Ability of a joint to maintain proper alignment during movement.

36. Kinesiology — Study of human movement mechanics.

37. Load Management — Regulation of physical stress placed on tissues during recovery.

38. Manual Therapy — Hands-on treatment techniques used to improve mobility.

39. Mobility Training — Exercises designed to improve movement efficiency.

40. Motor Control — Coordination of muscle activity to perform movements.

41. Neuromuscular Re-education — Techniques used to restore movement patterns after injury.

42. Occupational Demands — Physical requirements associated with specific job tasks.

43. Outcome Benchmark — Standard used to compare treatment progress.

44. Pain Modulation — Strategies used to reduce pain perception.

45. Patient Education — Instruction provided to improve self-management skills.

46. Performance Testing — Evaluation of strength, endurance, or agility.

47. Postural Control — Ability to maintain body alignment against gravity.

48. Progressive Loading — Gradually increasing resistance during rehabilitation.

49. Proprioception — Body's awareness of joint position and movement.

50. Referral Network — Professional connections used for coordinated patient care.

51. Rehabilitation Timeline — Expected stages of recovery after injury.

52. Resistance Training — Strength exercises using external resistance.

53. Return-to-Sport Criteria — Benchmarks used to determine readiness for athletic participation.

54. Risk Stratification — Classification of patients based on likelihood of complications.

55. Scar Tissue — Fibrous tissue that forms during healing.

56. Screening Assessment — Initial evaluation to identify potential conditions.

57. Sedentary Lifestyle — Pattern of minimal physical activity.

58. Soft Tissue Mobilization — Manual techniques applied to muscles and connective tissue.

59. Spasticity — Increased muscle tone resulting from neurological injury.

60. Stability Training — Exercises improving joint control during movement.

61. Strength Deficit — Reduced muscle force compared to expected levels.

62. Subacute Phase — Intermediate stage of injury recovery.

63. Symptom Management — Interventions aimed at reducing discomfort.

64. Therapeutic Alliance — Collaborative relationship between patient and clinician.

65. Therapeutic Modalities — Physical agents such as ultrasound or electrical stimulation.

66. Tissue Healing Phases — Biological stages of recovery after injury.

67. Treatment Frequency — Number of therapy sessions scheduled per week.

68. Treatment Tolerance — Patient ability to handle therapy intensity.

69. Unilateral Weakness — Muscle weakness affecting one side of the body.

70. Vestibular Rehabilitation — Therapy addressing balance and dizziness disorders.

71. Weight-Bearing Status — Physician-defined limits on limb loading.

72. Wellness Coaching — Guidance supporting long-term health habits.

73. Work Conditioning — Therapy preparing patients to return to job tasks.

74. Work Hardening — Intensive therapy simulating occupational demands.

75. Youth Athlete Development — Training programs supporting safe growth-related performance.

76. Activity Modification — Adjusting tasks to reduce injury risk.

77. Body Awareness — Conscious understanding of posture and movement.

78. Clinical Documentation — Written record of patient treatment and progress.

79. Deconditioning — Decline in physical fitness due to inactivity.

80. Dynamic Stretching — Movement-based flexibility exercises.

81. Exercise Prescription — Specific instructions for therapeutic exercise programs.

82. Functional Independence — Ability to perform activities without assistance.

83. Health Promotion — Strategies encouraging healthier lifestyle choices.

84. Injury Prevention — Programs designed to reduce injury risk.

85. Joint Mobilization — Manual therapy technique improving joint motion.

86. Load Tolerance — Maximum physical stress tissues can safely withstand.

87. Movement Screening — Evaluation identifying mobility limitations.

88. Musculoskeletal System — Bones, muscles, joints, and connective tissues.

89. Neural Mobility — Ability of nerves to move freely within surrounding tissues.

90. Orthotic Device — Brace used to support or align body structures.

91. Patient Compliance Barriers — Factors preventing adherence to treatment plans.

92. Performance Optimization — Strategies improving physical capability.

93. Progressive Overload — Gradual increase in exercise intensity.

94. Recovery Interval — Rest period between treatment sessions.

95. Rehabilitation Goal Setting — Establishing measurable treatment targets.

96. Strength Symmetry — Balanced muscle strength between body sides.

97. Therapeutic Progression — Advancement of treatment difficulty over time.

98. Treatment Outcome Tracking — Monitoring improvements across therapy sessions.

99. Wellness Maintenance — Ongoing health practices preventing recurrence of injury.

100. Work Capacity — Ability to perform sustained occupational activity.

Chapter 59

About the Author

Mason Preddy is the founder of Mason Maison™ Publishing and the creator of the *ScrubTales™* and *What Color Are Your Scrubs?™* career-alignment series, a growing body of work designed to help individuals make informed, sustainable decisions about entering and advancing within healthcare professions. His work focuses on the intersection of career alignment, workforce sustainability, and the long-term realities of healthcare practice, offering readers practical insight into the day-to-day experience of clinical roles rather than relying solely on traditional job descriptions and salary summaries.

Through the development of the *SCRUBfit™** career-alignment framework and the broader Mason's Alignment Theory (MAT), Mason's publications emphasize identity fit, role demands, workplace structure, and long-term career sustainability as essential factors in professional decision-making. His books are used by students, career changers, workforce development programs, and healthcare educators seeking clearer guidance on how individuals can find roles that match their strengths, values, and long-term lifestyle priorities.

Mason's mission is to help future and current healthcare professionals "find their fit before they commit," improving both individual career satisfaction and long-term retention across the healthcare workforce.

Chapter 60

Also by Mason Maison™ Publishing

What Color Are Your Scrubs?™

A comprehensive healthcare career guide exploring 345 current, emerging, and future roles across the healthcare workforce. Designed to help readers identify alignment between personality, strengths, lifestyle goals, and career pathways, this flagship resource introduces the *SCRUBfit™** career-alignment framework and Mason's Alignment Theory (MAT), offering structured tools to help students, career changers, and professionals make informed, sustainable decisions about entering healthcare.

ScrubTales™ Nurse Practitioner

A Real-World Career Guide That Tells the Truth About Responsibility, Identity, and Clinical Decision-Making

An in-depth exploration of the nurse practitioner profession, examining the cognitive demands, clinical accountability, compensation realities, and long-term sustainability considerations that shape advanced practice careers.

ScrubTales™ Physician Assistant

A Real-World Career Guide That Tells the Truth About Practicing Medicine Within a Team-Based System

A practical guide to the physician assistant profession, highlighting workflow realities, team-based decision-making structures, specialty mobility, and long-term career flexibility.

ScrubTales™ Registered Nurse

A Real-World Career Guide That Tells the Truth About the Demands and Tradeoffs of Nursing

An honest look at modern nursing practice, covering clinical expectations, workplace structures, emotional load, and the many pathways nurses use to evolve their careers over time.

ScrubTales™ Surgical Technologist

A Real-World Career Guide That Tells the Truth About the Operating Room and Surgical Teamwork

A behind-the-scenes examination of surgical team dynamics, sterile technique responsibilities, workflow intensity, and the precision-driven environment of operating room practice.

ScrubTales™ Diagnostic Medical Sonographer

A Real-World Career Guide That Tells the Truth About Diagnostic Imaging and Patient Care

A guide to the sonography profession exploring the technical skill, ergonomic demands, diagnostic responsibility, and patient interaction that define this specialized imaging career.

ScrubTales™ Respiratory Therapist

A Real-World Career Guide That Tells the Truth About Critical Care and Clinical Judgment

A deep look at respiratory therapy practice, focusing on high-acuity clinical environments, decision-making under pressure, and the evolving role of respiratory professionals across care settings.

Made in United States
Orlando, FL
05 November 2026

90231080R00174